# HOSPICE
# VOICES

# HOSPICE VOICES

## Lessons for Living at the End of Life

**Eric Lindner**

ROWMAN & LITTLEFIELD PUBLISHERS, INC.
Lanham • Boulder • New York • Toronto • Plymouth, UK

Published by Rowman & Littlefield Publishers, Inc.
A wholly owned subsidiary of
The Rowman & Littlefield Publishing Group, Inc.
4501 Forbes Boulevard, Suite 200, Lanham, Maryland 20706
www.rowman.com

10 Thornbury Road, Plymouth PL6 7PP, United Kingdom

Distributed by National Book Network

British Library Cataloguing in Publication Information Available

**Library of Congress Cataloging-in-Publication Data**

Lindner, Eric, 1958– author.
  Hospice voices : lessons for living at the end of life / Eric Lindner.
    p. ; cm.
  ISBN 978-1-4422-2059-1 (cloth : alk. paper)—ISBN 978-1-4422-2060-7
(electronic)
  I. Title.
  [DNLM: 1.  Hospice Care—Personal Narratives. 2.  Terminally Ill—
Personal Narratives. 3.  Attitude to Death—Personal Narratives. 4.  Sick
Role—Personal Narratives.  WB 310]
  RT87.T45
  362.17'560922—dc23                                    2013015719

⊗™ The paper used in this publication meets the minimum requirements of
American National Standard for Information Sciences—Permanence of Paper
for Printed Library Materials, ANSI/NISO Z39.48-1992.

Printed in the United States of America

to Ellen

for everything

All book profits will be donated to organizations committed to improving the lives of hospice patients and their families, such as the George Washington Institute for Spirituality & Health (Washington, D.C.), Hospice of Central New York (Liverpool), Hospice Support of Fauquier County (Virginia), Johns Hopkins Medicine (Baltimore), Kaua'i Hospice, St. Joseph Mercy Hospice (Ann Arbor, Michigan), St. Mary's Hospice (Leonardtown, Maryland), and other entities, including those listed at www.hospicevoices.com.

# CONTENTS

# PREFACE

I wasn't sure what to expect from Bob Zimmerman. But I sure didn't expect this from my first hospice patient: some of the most fun I've ever had, and best advice I've ever received.

The Ohioan joins a Native American from central California, a Neapolitan from Texas (by way of Brooklyn's Little Italy), and four Virginia natives. I'm assigned many more than seven patients, but it just so happens that what Bob, Little One, Dolly, Gordon, Ellen, Howard, and Cricket have to say helps me navigate some choppiness in my own life. It also just so happens that they're the most fascinating people I've ever met.

As regards the definition of *fascinating*, I consider myself a fairly strict constructionist. I've fought bulls beside a drunken matador in Avila, interviewed homicidal gang members at the behest of my Nobel laureate professor in Chicago, negotiated with even scarier-looking oligarchs in Moscow, wolfed naan with a no-carb Hollywood actress in Mumbai, and schmoozed with U.S. presidents in my hometown of Washington. Fascinating though many of my pre-hospice experiences were, I wouldn't trade a single one for a single hour as a "companion caregiver."

During my volunteer orientation, I'm told that the average hospice patient survives three months. Once out in the field, however, I learn that there's no such thing as an "average hospice patient." Every patient is unique. Some of mine thrive for years—fighting every step of the way. Others slip away in hours—laughing as they depart.

In contemporary society, famous voices are ubiquitous, and so often boring, whereas the voices of the common folk are inspiring but muzzled. This book lets them speak for a change.

Given their blindness, bedpans, breathing tubes, and chemotherapy, of course my patients comprehend their fearsome, depressing mortality. But they don't want my pity. Just my ear.

It has at times been a challenge translating their voices into printed words. For starters, I didn't volunteer with any intention of writing anything, so it wasn't until well into my hospice work that I gave any thought to gathering and preserving "source material." But by then many of my patients had died. Once the notion of a book had taken root, I was determined, first, not to let it interfere with my privilege to serve, and, second, to chronicle as a friend, not in the manner of a clinician or journalist. So, for instance, fearing its use might be intrusive, chilling, or otherwise counterproductive to my cardinal mission of simply being present with and for my patients and their loved ones, I decided against the use of a digital recorder (openly, let alone covertly).

Despite such constraints, the following stories are factual. My job as research assistant to a prolific, meticulous legal scholar taught me a thing or two about being methodical and attentive to detail. As I had to submit a report on each patient visit, this book's methodology is anchored upon hundreds of such submissions. However, as the short, clinical nature of the reports omitted many memorable quotes and subtle details, I also consulted my original notes, typically scribbled down as soon as I'd hopped into my car, while the recollections were still fresh in my mind. Patients, their family members, hospice colleagues, and others with knowledge or expertise kindly provided an additional check on veracity and context: reviewing draft manuscripts, and offering a host of valuable corrections and suggestions. (But all errors and omissions are mine alone.) Finally, unlike most hospice accounts—which fictionalize identities—the vast majority of my characters are real people, related to whom I've received written consent to name names. Consequently, you'll come to know real patients, their real families, their real living situations and coping strategies, and my very real (albeit well-intentioned) bungling as a novice caregiver.

I hope you'll forgive my mistakes, remember their names—and never forget their voices.

Shared joy is a double joy;
shared sorrow is half a sorrow.

—Swedish proverb

# AN APTLY NAMED CAREGIVER

Joy LeBaron seems really nice but distracted. "I'd love to have another volunteer . . . Eric—did you say your name was?" The executive director of Hospice Support of Fauquier County (Virginia), Inc., is a slight woman. She looks about five to ten years younger than me, so in her early to mid-forties. She also looks unpretentious: her ensemble of slacks, blouse, and cable-knit sweater is loose fitting; her short hair, simply cut, is a wavy, bang-heavy lattice of several shades of blonde. Though she clearly appreciates my walking in off the street in February 2009, its not being on her to-do list is mildly disruptive; if, that is, it's possible to disrupt the disruption that governs Joy's feng shui. Her small office is crammed with collapsed walkers and wheelchairs, stands of green oxygen tanks, a cluttered conference table, an overflowing bookcase. It smells musty. The coffee at the base of the pot looks carbonized. The phone rings a lot, kicking over to voicemail. "I've currently got twenty patients. I could add another twenty by the end of the day—if I had more volunteers. I can't give my patients anywhere near the hours they want."

According to the National Hospice and Palliative Care Organization (NHPCO), her overburdened not-for-profit is one of 5,300 in the United States—quite a rate of growth, considering America's first hospice didn't open until 1974, in New Haven, Connecticut (in association with Yale University). Circa 2013, more than half the world's hospices are located in the United States.

Joy's an expert in "palliative care," of which hospice is the best-known paradigm. Such care is all about comforting, not curing. Of those who die every year in the United States, nearly one in two are served by hospice. Moreover, as patients—and their loved ones—generally rate their experiences very favorably, and the per diem hospice cost is but a tiny fraction of the per diem hospital cost, hospice is a very bright component in the oft-maligned U.S. healthcare system. One reason hospice is so efficient has to do with the role played by volunteers, nearly 500,000 of whom serve 1,650,000 terminally ill patients, annually. At many hospices, the volunteers outnumber the paid professionals.

"Okay, then. So I've come to the right place. Throw me into the hopper."

Suddenly I'm not there, as Joy's hand shoots to her mouth, and she spins around. "Hhh! Where'd I put that? . . ." But then she remembers me. "Sorry . . ."

"I'm sorry. I should have called first."

"No, no. I'm glad you stopped in. It's just that . . . you need orientation, and training."

"Fair enough. When's your next session?"

"See, that's just it. We're so small, we've not got anything lined up right now. We're strapped for funds. The financial crisis dried up our donor base. But," she adds, "I'll e-mail Rosalie Palermo at Haymarket Hospice. They're much bigger. Unlike us, they get funds from Medicare as well as from Virginia, Maryland, and the District of Columbia. Rosalie has new volunteer sessions all the time. She has to."

"Where are they based?"

Her head cants, she smiles. "Haymarket."

"Gosh, what a dumb question. 'Course."

"They've got maybe a thousand volunteers! Plus a paid professional staff of seven hundred or so."

"That does sound big."

"Once you're trained in Haymarket, you'd be on my roster, too. We often share patients."

## MARCH–MAY 2009

Joy follows through on her promise, and I exchange e-mails with Rosalie. Haymarket Hospice does hold regular orientation and training sessions; however, I'm often out of town.

Still, I fill out some forms and coax some friends into submitting reference letters. (Asked to attest that I'm no psychopath, several hesitate.) Meanwhile, Rosalie puts me in touch with existing caregivers, both volunteers and paid professionals. "We find it often helps," she says, "to hear why others are doing it and how reality does—and/or doesn't—differ from what they felt might be the case coming in." I reach out to her referrals, and learn a lot.

## JUNE 2

6:23 P.M. My first orientation session is well under way in a converted antebellum Virginia office building of fieldstone, brick, milk-painted plaster, and lovely heart-of-pine, where, 148 Junes prior, a then-unknown lemon-sucking fanatical Presbyterian preacher named Thomas Jackson was en route to rescue Confederate general P. G. T. Beauregard at First Bull Run—earning his nickname in the process: Stonewall. I can't figure out how to buzz myself in using the after-hours intercom contraption. After several frustrating minutes, Rosalie rescues me.

Trapped within the vestibule, I hear the elevator ding. She flies out and charges over, the rush of air billowing her purple blouse. "I hope this isn't a test," I say. "It is," says she. "But I grade on a curve!" "Sorry I'm late," I add. "No worries!" she responds. We swap smiles and shake hands, which rattles and clanks her chunky silver necklace, hoop earrings, and bracelets. Black bell-bottomed pants and pink ballet-flat shoes complete a sort of happy hippy ensemble.

We head down into the cool basement, where I join three other prospective volunteers around a big, gleaming table. We wave, say hi to each other. Clockwise from my right, there's a thin, fidgety, frail-looking man whom I'd guess to be in his early thirties, in baggy grass-stained jodhpurs, an older, smiling señora in a floral blouse, and

a dapper gentleman in natty herringbone, who I'm told once ran with
Dean Martin and other members of The Rat Pack. The coffee smells
good, and the cookies look tempting. The softly playing New Age music is soothing, but, as the bright overhead lights aren't, I tug my cap
low over my brow, shielding my sensitive eyes.

While we recruits sign in, settle in, sip, and nosh, Rosalie remains
standing at the end of the table. "There may be one or two more strag-
glers, but I think this is probably it."

Rosalie's smile dominates her personality. Though expansive and
expressive, it can't contain—or communicate—the full extent of her
ebullience, even when abetted by her halogen hazel eyes. In toto, it's
the pardoning countenance of a Been There, Done That woman, of a
mother of two boys, one girl, and the ex-wife of a man who skipped
town just after she'd delivered his son. Her naturally curly auburn hair
is now crazily spirally so, as a result of chemo. In a Boston accent she
says, "Please raise your hand if, during the past year, you've either experienced the loss of a loved one or you're currently caring for someone
who's terminally ill."

All hands go up except mine, sending a few glances my way. Like
Rosalie, whose mother received hospice care until her death in 2002,
everyone else in the room, via brief summaries, explains how they've
been positively touched by hospice and, thus, wants to "give forward."

But my motivations are atypical, and my path to this conference room
is anything but linear. It follows decades of discursive dabbling, from a
few weeks in a hospital burn unit to nine years on the board of a big
university. All told, as a volunteer I've done some good and screwed
some things up. At fifty, with my second of two kids having just shipped
off to college, and my business on cruise control, the restlessness that's
always bubbled beneath the surface of my life is no longer masked by
the film of details attendant to earning a living and raising a family. But
being restive isn't my only motivation. Most of my patients would be
seniors, and I've always been attracted to "wise elders." My wife closes
the sale. When I ask Ellen what she thinks of my spending ten hours a
week providing companion care for a revolving door of terminal illness,
she replies, "It's something not many people can do, but I do think you
have what it takes and should give it a try."

The "why volunteer?" responses of my fellow trainees don't tell me much, but they're suggestive. Everyone seems a bit diffident and/or tired, like it's been a long day, illness, or both. Rosalie's referrals had shed more particulars on what I might be getting myself into.

My favorite motivational story is that of Gil Booker, Joy's assistant. Having been diagnosed with kidney cancer at age forty-three, Gil was two days away from surgery when his doctor suddenly called it off.

"Off??" Gil exclaims. "Why?"

The oncologist explained how, notwithstanding all the consistent and encouraging images of a shrinking kidney mass, out of nowhere, the latest scan showed robust bone cancer. "It's metastasized surprisingly fast." Pointing to bright spots in the skull, ribs, and elsewhere on the image, the oncologist explained that surgery—any type of remediation—was now, unfortunately, hopeless. Consequently, the doctor strongly advised Gil to forego the planned removal of the kidney mass and, instead, get his will in order, draft up a Bucket List, and wring out as much enjoyment as he can, "until it becomes too much." (Bone cancer is excruciatingly painful.)

Naturally, Gil was in shock. Naturally, once home, he and his wife hugged a lot, cried a lot. Less naturally, Gil ignored his oncologist and insisted on going ahead with the scheduled surgery. The result? In addition to successfully removing the kidney tumor, several bone biopsies reveal that there was in fact no bone cancer. "We can't explain it!" the oncologist exclaimed. "We don't know what those bright lights on the imaging were!" Gil's been a hospice volunteer ever since, for twenty-five years.

I'm thinking of Gil as Rosalie passes around a sign-in sheet, along with troves of information, a small pile for each prospect. It's hardly light reading, what with book, pamphlet, monograph, and one-page handout titles like "Good Mourning," "Infection Control," "Hazardous Materials–Management Program," "101 Things to Do with a Person Who Has Alzheimer's Disease," and, in the event of suspected patient abuse, "Confidential Occurrence Report."

"I know this is a lot of information," says Rosalie. "But please read it all, when you get a chance. The most important information is the list of *Dos* and *Don'ts* in that purple-bound book there, titled *Student Manual*.

"*Dos*," she explains, "like being dependable. Being genuine." *Do listen. Do keep good boundaries*, both physical and philosophical, such as religion. *Do encourage a life review. Do be comfortable with quiet*; "silence is okay." *Do remember to care for yourself, and to communicate with the volunteer manager/hospice team*, both in regular written reports and, if necessary, by telephone call, if something's in need of more urgent attention. *Do remember that little things mean a lot*; "what you give is immeasurable." Finally, as tragic and sickening as this sounds, by all means, *do report signs of abuse*.

"Meanwhile, on the flip side, *don't visit your patient if you're ill*." *Don't play doctor or nurse*, either by offering advice or dispensing any sort of medication. *Don't judge*; "especially *don't try to referee a family squabble!*" *Don't break confidentiality. Don't give unsolicited advice*; here again, religion often comes into play. *Don't take on more patients than you can manage. Don't take it personally*—whatever. "*Don't expect your patient to conform to your standards/expectations.*" *Don't interrupt when the patient is sharing*. "And, last but not least, *don't assume you know what their needs/feelings are.*"

"That's all?" says a prospect, voicing the reaction of us all.

Rosalie nods, and smiles. "I know. It's a lot. But, first, as to the reporting, we don't expect much. Just the basics, anything noteworthy. Nobody likes paperwork. More generally, it boils down to one thing, really: being compassionate. Compassion trumps everything. As those of you who've suffered through a loss—or who are now suffering—know, I'd wager. I am very sorry for what you've gone through, or are going through now. I hope I might, maybe, offer you some tools to ease your suffering.

"Thank you, all of you, for your willingness to volunteer. There's such an enormous need out there."

According to NHPCO, each year nearly five hundred thousand volunteers rack up a total of twenty million hours. This translates into less than an hour a week; most patients are looking for three to five hours, if not more. Haymarket Hospice boasts "nearly 1,500 patient contacts each and every day." However, thin volunteer ranks mean many such "patient contacts" are no more than five-minute phone calls. "I'm not complaining!" Rosalie is quick to note. "I understand, totally! We all have such busy lives . . . our own bundle of existing commitments, obligations, and other priorities. But, still . . ."

The volunteer shortage is tragic in two ways. First, about two-thirds of America's terminally ill die in hospitals or nursing homes, as opposed to in their own home (or the home of a loved one), where nearly nine in ten would prefer to die. Second, the last emotion hundreds of thousands of Americans experience is—loneliness. "Being lonely at the end of life is so sad, so tragic. I've heard it—loneliness—called the most desperate of all English words. And it's far worse in most other countries.

"But let's not dwell on a downer, right? Once we're through with our nine hours of orientation and training, and you're out in the field, I'm confident that, like almost all volunteers report, you're going to experience something truly special, a real win-win. In addition to helping others, and despite the unavoidable sadness, you'll be helping yourself, too, by discovering a sublime sense of fulfillment. I know it! I've every confidence you'll feel as I do: helping people at this stage of their lives feel less alone is a real privilege.

"Now . . . a bit about me. I've been around the block!"

I'll say. By the sound of it, she's just about seen it all: miraculous recoveries, abrupt deaths; selfless doting by strangers, shocking abandonment by supposed loved ones; warm collegiality among hospice workers, stymying by higher-ups in a cold corporate bureaucracy. "I need to warn you," Rosalie cautions, "we've got nearly seven hundred paid staff and a thousand volunteers interacting with terminally ill patients more than a thousand times each day . . ." She shakes her head. "At times, just the HIPAA requirements—"

She pauses, in response to several puzzled stares. "Sorry. HIPAA stands for the Health Insurance Portability and Accountability Act. It's a mouthful, I know. You'll be able to read all about it, in your packet."

"Oh," says the man in the grass-stained jodhpurs.

"What I was getting at is that, sometimes, wanting to be compassionate conflicts with needing to be legally compliant. Now, sometimes, I think the view from the front lines—from you guys—makes a lot more sense than what the armchair quarterbacks have to say, back in there." She wags her head toward the warren of offices beyond the recently tuck-pointed stone walls.

"But I don't want to blow things out of proportion, either. There are a lot of good people in executive management. And, like at most places, they often got there by working themselves up through the ranks. Many

have far more experience than me. I've only been doing this for about
a year, drawn by how much help it was to my mom, and me, during her
last weeks, and months, in oh-two.

"I bring something else to the table, too. I'm a cancer survivor. I
thought I'd bought the farm." Rosalie looks around, prompting several
knowing nods.

"But, we'll all buy the farm, some day. As everyone from Buddha to
Ben Franklin has remarked, we all have a terminal condition. It's called
being human!

"We pretty much all begin the same, as a former midwife now on
staff will tell you. It's more our endings that vary, like the seven hundred thousand Americans who die each year of heart disease versus
the seventy thousand Alzheimer's claims. Hmm . . ." An index finger
taps her lower lip. "Ten hearts for every one mind. Fodder for a poet,
if you ask me.

"So . . . terminal illness, which seems such a concrete, finite, hard-
edged term, is actually somewhat slippery. Though it depends on semantics, it really boils down to two things: First, that our time-related
frame of reference shifts, from the flipping of calendar pages to the
ticking of a stopwatch. Second, that our cause of death appears rea-
sonably predictable. However, as you get some experience under your
belts, you'll begin to see the wiggle room in both of these terms, too—
reasonable and predictable. For instance, Medicare will only reimburse
Haymarket Hospice if two conditions exist. First, the patient must have
given up trying to seek a cure. Second, a doctor must say that the patient
is not expected to last longer than six months.

"But I'll share with you two little hospice secrets. Treasures, really.
First, we in hospice like to say that, between the curing of and caring for
patients, there's plenty of room for healing—of human beings. Second,
for every six patients that America's five thousand–plus hospices took in
last year, one was discharged—alive!

"Now, admittedly, most live discharges involve transfer to a hospital's ER, ICU, or some other form of more intensive acute care prior
to death. However, for a significant number of people, things don't get
worse—they get better. In other words, once they formally renounce all
efforts at finding a cure, BINGO! lots get cured, somehow. Many live
for years. Decades.

"A friend of mine, a fertility specialist, reports a similar phenomenon. He tells me that he can't remember the number of times that couples—once they've resigned themselves to the so-called fact that they can't conceive, and opt for adoption—suddenly can, and do conceive. Isn't life great, sometimes?

"I know you already know this: what you're about to undertake can involve some very dark days and depressing moments. But know this, too: it's often darkest before the dawn.

"Once we're through with all four of our sessions, you'll receive one of these." She holds up a framed certificate that reads, "In recognition of successful completion of the Volunteer Patient/Family Care Training Program."

## JUNE 4 AND 9

I make two more sessions, but, away on travel, I miss the fourth and final one. I watch the DVD, at home.

## JULY 6

Well before my certificate arrives, Rosalie phones me. "Ready??"

"We'll see," I reply.

"Okay, then! I've got your first patient. You're going to love him! Let me brief you . . ."

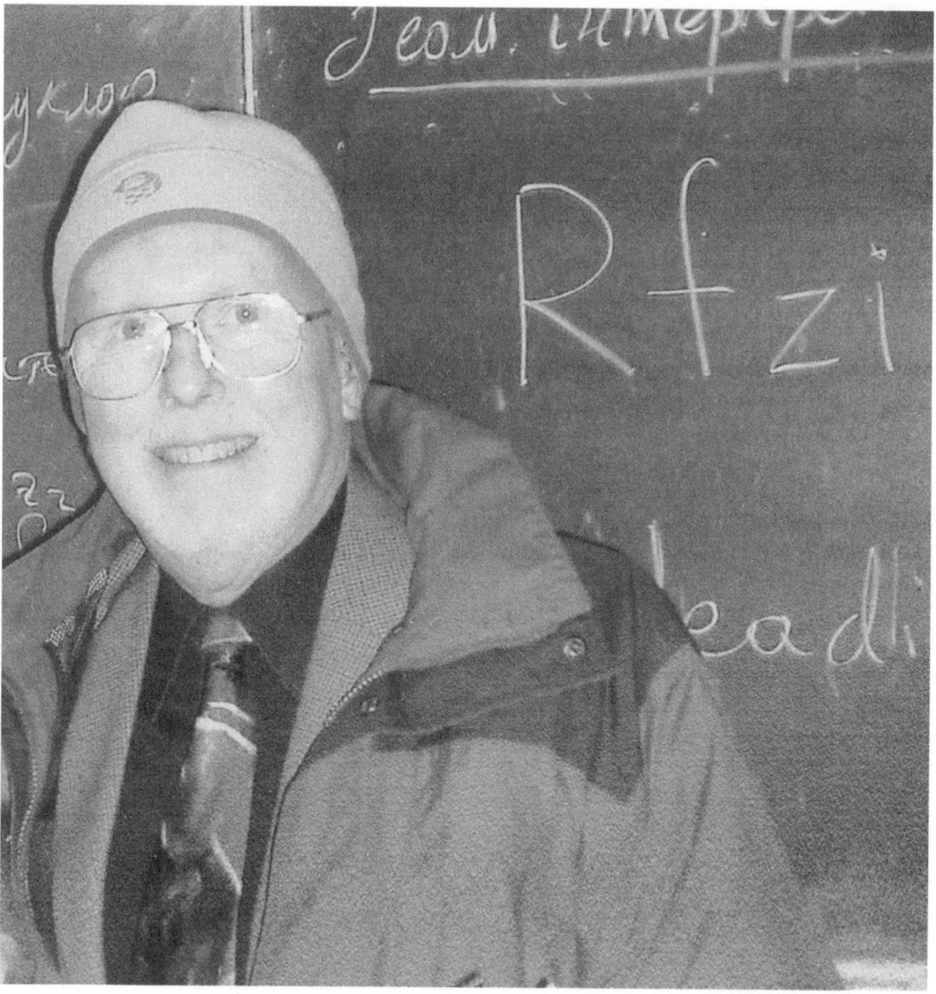
Rfzi

# FIND THE KEY THAT
# UNLOCKS EMPATHY

**B**ob Zimmerman is seventy-three, white, and a native Ohioan. He earned his BA in international affairs from the University of Akron. After personally witnessing JFK's famous call to peaceful arms, Bob joined the Peace Corps and headed to the Philippines. After his two-year tour, he joined the U.S. State Department's Agency for International Development (AID), related to which he spent years in Thailand, Indonesia, and Egypt. (While at State, in between travel, Bob earned his MA and PhD from American University, also in international affairs.) Bob then tackled various NGO jobs, all of which blended education, community outreach, public-private partnership, and economic development. For instance, he escorted tens of thousands of young students on "working tours" of the federal government (an institution of which he's incredibly proud, even though he wrote a book cataloguing its waste). His final career stop was as a Fulbright Scholar, teaching political science and international affairs to college students at Tavrida University in Ukraine. He's fluent in six languages. Spiritually inquisitive his entire life, he grew up a Congregationalist, dabbled in Buddhism, Jainism, and other belief systems, converted to Catholicism to marry his Filipina wife, and, in the past few years, has loved listening to the soothing sermons of his daughter, Jenny, who, along with her copastoring and much more pyrotechnic husband, Mark, evangelizes on behalf of Jesus at River Church, sharing a small strip mall with a Flooring America outlet in Winchester, Virginia. Bob lives with Jenny's younger sister, Kathleen. Six months prior, Kathleen had insisted her dad move in with her, from the condo he'd lived in for fifteen years on King Street in Alexandria, about ten miles south of the Capitol.

"Bob moved," Rosalie tells me, "because his cancer'd returned. It first presented in his prostate, in 1999. Radiation plus chemo drove it into remission, but now it's back, with a vengeance. It's metastasized throughout his body. Then there's the Alzheimer's . . . Yet he's undaunted. Always cheerful. Whenever he and I talk, in between his growing lapses and non sequiturs, he speaks with a rare clarity. It lifts my spirits."

Though divorced, Bob's relationship with his ex-wife has always remained warm and respectful. His daughters have given him four grandchildren, three of which are boys. His siblings include two sisters, Betsy and Jan (they live a ways away), and one younger brother, Jack, with whom Bob's especially close and who also lives in Virginia, an hour from Kathleen (two, if traffic's bad), near Bob's former Alexandria condo.

Bob loved running marathons (past tense), especially the New York City Marathon, even though he lost all ten toenails while recording his best time of just over three hours. He still loves to swim, though he's rarely able, and paint, which he does nearly every day. His medium is watercolor, and his favorite subject is nature, especially flowers and his beloved birch tree—to him what the sunset was to van Gogh, the hay bale to Wyeth.

"Know what I think he most loves?" asks Rosalie. "Simply being around people, so he can infect them with his sunny optimism. I mean, he's been bugging me for weeks to place someone with him. I think you and he will be a perfect match."

Rosalie always tries to conclude her briefings with at least one item from the patient's Bucket List and suggest how the caregiver might help make it happen. "Bob really wants to travel one last time to Canada, with Jack. They'd swing by their sister's, then head up to his family's lakeside cabin, which he so enjoyed growing up. Bob calls it his own personal slice of heaven. However, the odds of his making the trip aren't looking so good."

## JULY 9–10, 2009

But Bob sure sounds good when he and I first talk. "That's *great!*" he hollers into the phone, when I offer to visit him from time to time, pitching relief for Kathleen, Jenny, and Jack. "I'm *so* excited!"

I have difficulty processing the disconnect of Bob's elation—and imminent death. I wonder what's going on inside his head, if he's trying to make himself more appealing to me by not appearing a downer, whatever. I wonder, too, if he's doped up somehow, as his high-as-a-kite ebullience reminds me of some of my friends when they're under the influence of ganja.

"Any idea what you'd like to do, Bob, when I visit? So I come prepared?"

"I want pancakes."

"Pancakes?"

"Yep. See, while undergoing radiation and chemo, I couldn't taste anything. Now I'm off 'em? My taste is back. It's great! And the first thing I want to taste is pancakes.

"But, now, with my memory going, who knows whether by this evening I'll even remember what they tasted like! So we'd better move fast! Plus, my weight's dropped from one seventy one, to one thirty one. If I'm going to run another marathon, I need to add some weight."

The chances of Bob running another marathon are extremely remote. Though I try to hide it, my tonal skepticism is detected by the gifted linguist. "You'll see, Eric. You'll see."

The following day, I arrive at the home of Bob's daughter, just across Bull Run creek. I'm not a naturally nervous guy, but my nerves are sure amped up now as I pull alongside the curb outside Kathleen's home and park. While walking toward the front door, I reflect on the fact that I might really suck at this and wonder what mysterious hand nudged me toward this particular expression of community service.

Your garden-variety upper-middle-class Northern Virginia home, circa the early twenty-first century, on maybe a quarter of an acre of land, Kathleen's place is surrounded by scores like it, all somewhat similar but also somewhat unique. One distinctive feature is the stack on the porch of unused lawn signs advertising the construction company

Kathleen and her husband own and operate, which, like so many in the area, has been clobbered by the housing crash.

I knock. She opens the door. We shake hands. "Hi," she says, "nice to meet you." "Nice to meet you," I say. Very attractive, she's about 5'7", fit, and tan. "Dad's having a rough day."

Right on cue, Bob emerges up through a door to the basement and steps over to meet me. "Hello!" He extends his hand, which I shake. He sandwiches my hand with his other hand, peers into my eyes, and smiles. Though about the same height as his daughter, he's a lot less healthy looking. Whereas her clothes are chic and form-fitting, his are baggy, frumpy. His khakis are rumpled, his running shoes scuffed. Unlike her auburn tresses, the chemo's dispensed with most of his light-brown hair. "Thank you for agreeing to spend some time with me. I think I'm about beginning to wear out my welcome here." He winks at Kathleen.

Kathleen looks aghast. "Dad! Never!"

Releasing one of his hands from mine, he brushes her cheek. "I know," he coos.

He and I say goodbye to Kathleen, and head off. Outside, on the way to my car, we pass some daisies, bursting with color. Bob pauses, cups one, bends over, and sniffs. He turns to me and beams. "I think each flower is a smile from God."

"What a wonderful notion."

"Okay if we run by my optometrist first? Fell, broke my glasses. It shouldn't take long."

"My time's your time." Only now do I notice the cuts on his chin and elbow and the bruising on the back of his hands. I see this sort of thing all the time with my dad, who's eighty-three to Bob's seventy-three.

While waiting for his glasses on a bench inside the shop, Bob notices my red, swollen eye. "Hurt your eye?"

"Long story: Fifteen operations over fifteen years. Most recently a cornea transplant. My eye's not sure it likes the alien intruder. But I don't want to bore you."

"I'm sorry. Actually—I'm not. It happened for a reason. Everything does. Problems are opportunities. For instance, I'm blind in my left eye." This Bob says with less apparent regret than had he said, "I prefer Pepsi, but all they had was Coke."

"Gosh! I didn't know. Sorry." I slump at the pettiness of my own problems.

"It was a blessing, I tell you, the early onset of this half-full glass. It set me up for life."

"A blessing??"

"Uh-huh. My best friend did it to me. Pushed me down a hill, on a toboggan. I slammed straight into a tree. I was ten."

"Oh, man. Your friend must've felt awful!"

"He did. But it was a blessing: an opportunity for Providence to fill my half-full glass."

"I'm all ears. All . . . eye."

"Hah! So, some twelve years later, I'm this young man. Full of piss and vinegar, but clueless as to what I want to do, or . . . should do in life. Then I happen to hear President Kennedy's famous speech about the creation of the Peace Corps."

"I've seen the footage, plenty of times. 'Ask not what your country can do for you—'"

"'—but what you can do for your country.' Exactly! So, I answer his rallying cry and join the Peace Corps. They send me to the Philippines. Two years later, I'm at State, which turns me right back around and ships me off to Vietnam, in sixty-seven, as part of its Chiêu Hồi Program. It means *open arms* in Vietnamese. Beautiful language. Beautiful people."

"Your Vietnamese pretty good?"

Bob nods. "Lord knows I've been saddled with a few liabilities. But for every one, I've also been blessed with several assets. A facility with languages is one such asset."

Turns out he has a photographic memory, which helps to explain his fluency in Thai, Tagalog, Vietnamese, Indonesian, and Russian. "Languages are joyous presents to be unwrapped," he concludes.

"So, what'd you do in . . . Open Arms?"

"I opened some eyes instead."

Bob talks about how the Vietcong would appear in a flash, wreak mayhem—then vanish through the thick brush or via trap-doored tunnels; of how everyone got paranoid, not knowing which smiling villagers were friend or foe. Bob's mission was to win over the hearts and minds of the locals, to help the United States win the PR war with the Chinese. It seemed a tall order.

Now his order's tall—for real.

As I look around for Bob's glasses repairman, wondering when we might be able to hit McDonald's, our primary mission, Bob gets to the point of his parable. "One day, a group of locals emerges from the jungle. Everyone in camp's on edge, for though the Vietcong weren't into the wearing of explosive vests, et cetera, they were very cagey. These locals might be Vietcong, or they might be friendlies. If Vietcong, this group might just be diversionary, to allow another group to mount a flanking operation.

"At the head of this group of six is an especially tough-looking guy. Short, ropy. Though I'm no military man, even I can tell he's undertaking recon, counting our tents, personnel, et cetera. Clearly, he's the leader. But, lo and behold, in his open arms—ha!—he's carrying a small boy. Maybe ten, the same age I was when I lost my eye. His eye's a mess, too."

"What a coincidence!"

"Yes. If, that is, you believe in coincidence.

"Anyway, though the Green Berets had made it perfectly clear that we were to keep our distance, something gets hold of me. So I blow past the Green Berets and head for the boy.

"The Green Beret captain goes nuts. 'What do you think you're doing, Zimmerman?!'

"'My job,' I say.

"'And what's that?'

"'Trying to win hearts and minds.'

"'But we don't know if these guys are Charlie or not. This might all just be a ruse to scope out our position.'

"'That's the funny thing about hearts and minds, Captain. There's always some risk of being hurt.'"

To his credit, the officer doesn't stop Bob. Though not yet fluent, Bob's Vietnamese is good enough for him to comprehend that the father had come to see if his boy's eye could be fixed. "And?" I wonder.

Bob shakes his head. "Poor thing. It's obvious the boy's in tremendous pain, but he's being so brave, so stoic. Like dogs, you know? When they're in pain? Like it's their duty not to complain to their master?"

Bob persuades the captain to allow the medic to inject morphine into the boy's arm and clean and bandage the eye. Bob relates the bad news that the boy's eye is probably beyond repair, "But we can try." The father hoists his son as one of his lieutenants accepts the narcotics, cream, gauze, tape, etc., from Bob. "Thus far, the dad's not made a sound, not a peep of thanks or otherwise. But, as he heads off, his eyes thank me. And I notice from the way he's favoring one of his own eyes, the way I'd learned to do also, since being blinded, that it's not just the son who's got an eye problem. The dad does, too."

"'Hold up!'" Bob says, in Vietnamese. He walks over and peers into the father's eyes. "As I thought, the dad's got cataracts. In both eyes. I point at my own eyes, then the dad's, one after the other. 'Return. Tomorrow. With your son. Can help you.'

"The father's noncommittal. He studies me. Glances at his boy. Exchanges looks with his lieutenant. Meanwhile, as he'd not authorized the offer I've just extended—of our medic performing two eye operations—the Green Beret is fuming. Berating me with an evil-eye stare.

"The father clearly heard me, but he doesn't acknowledge the fact. He simply turns and leads his group away, me wondering if I'll ever see this guy again or if, in some way, I've just put American lives in jeopardy, the dad being angry at my telling him we couldn't save his boy's eye."

A few days later, father and son return to take Bob up on his out-of-line offer. Unfortunately, the boy loses his eye. "Poor, brave thing," says Bob.

"And the father?" I wonder.

"The medic operates on both eyes."

"Successful?"

"Maybe the most successful eye operations performed throughout the course of the war." Two weeks after the operations, the father returns for another visit. This time, the men bring along their weapons, held high above their heads, nozzles affixed with white scraps signifying not just surrender but the formation of a new alliance. "They tell me it's one of the largest, if not the largest, crossovers during the entire war."

"Here's to Operation Open Arms," I say, hoisting an imaginary champagne flute.

Bob plays along, smiling. "To Operation Open Arms."

"Courtesy of Bob Zimmerman."

Bob shakes his head. "No. Courtesy of my friend who blinded me. Thereby allowing me, for the first time, to really see what empathy's all about."

As the optometrist arrives with the optimist's repaired glasses, I reflect on my lesson. It humbles me. In the span of fifteen minutes, free of charge, Bob teaches me more than have some of the world's leading scholars over the course of many years, costing loads of money.

After settling the repaired eyewear on the bridge of his nose, Bob inquires, "How much do I owe you?"

"Not a penny," says the optometrist.

"Why, thank you," says Bob.

As the kind man heads off to serve another customer, Bob turns to me. "Pancake time!"

"Wanna hit Frost Diner?" I ask. "Down in Warrenton? It has amazing pancakes. There's also an IHOP in Warrenton. And I love just about anything at Cracker Barrel in Manassas."

"Thanks, but I like McDonald's pancakes just fine. And it's just around the corner."

"Mickey D's it is, then."

Once at The Golden Arches, Bob slides into a booth. I head over to place his order.

I return with his food and sit across from him. The smells cascade into one another: my hot coffee, his sticky syrup, the sausage and its mystery meat. As Bob peels back the OJ container's thin seal, an escaping spritz splatters his new spectacles—prompting a chuckle.

He cleans his lenses and sets to work on the first sausage link. He's methodical. Tearing open a packet of ketchup, applying it evenly. Carving the dappled gray cylinder, spearing it, inserting it into his mouth. Chewing and swallowing languidly, nostalgically. Once the first link is history, he turns his attention to the pancakes. First slathering on a soft pat of butter, then drowning them in two packets of syrup. Every other bite chased by some OJ.

His repast concludes with a final slurp, which triggers a belch. "Excuse me. Ahh," he adds, patting his belly, as his flung plastic fork clatters against the Styrofoam plate. "Now I'm ready for that Marine Corps Marathon! This is the sort of thing that made it all worthwhile."

"It?"

"My refusing to quit. Refusing to accept the 'unanimous diagnosis.' My experience has been, if something's unanimous, then you know there's something wrong with it. Something—fundamental—that everyone fails to see."

And off Bob goes on another parable of vision, or lack thereof. Of how, at the first appearance of cancer, every doctor said he was a goner. But he refused to quit. He hoped, questioned, searched, and prodded . . . until he came across some promising oncology research. The treatment was radical, unapproved by the FDA. "It was no picnic. Trust me. But my PSA plummets, and I go into full remission."

"Wow!"

"But the Big C's back after almost ten years. This time around, however, I'm all out of medical options. But I'm not throwing in the towel. God's got the towel. I trust Him fully."

## JULY 16

Having learned about Bob's recent trip to Kiev, whence I'd returned a few months prior, I feel he'd enjoy meeting my friend George Woloshyn, a sixty-seven-year-old former FEMA inspector general born in Ukraine. While planning lunch over the phone, Bob's his typical ebullient self.

When I arrive to collect him, Kathleen opens the door. She's subdued. "Hi. I'll go get Dad."

With her gone, I wander around. The home's clean, airy, sunny, pine-scented, with a medley of those inspirational plaques and posters quoting Rilke and Franklin that one finds at Cracker Barrel. A fit-looking boy and girl blow past me, half-dressed in soccer outfits. As the boy pauses to give me the up-down, I notice his ten-year-old six-pack. His sister's a bit older but just as fit. Backing up carefully, so these balls of energy don't knock me over and damage my recently implanted artificial hips, I turn around to find myself face-to-face with Kathleen's husband, who's on the phone at his desk in his home office. He's blond, rugged looking, with an air of stoicism, and built like the Hulk. (This I can tell just from his torso and neck.) From the snatches of conversation I overhear (without trying to eavesdrop), he doesn't sound like a happy camper. Few in the construction trade are in July 2009.

Just then Bob steps onto the first-floor landing from his basement apartment and shuffles over to meet me. Kathleen gives him a hug and says, "Have fun!" but he hardly seems to notice or care.

I glance at Kathleen. My chipper tone dissembles. "Back in a couple hours, I imagine."

Twenty minutes later, Bob, George, and I are sitting at a table in front of a stone fireplace at the Brass Cannon Restaurant. "Bob," I say, "I just thought it was such a neat coincidence that you'd spent so much time in Ukraine, I'd recently been there, and George was born there. I thought you guys, especially, could really swap some stories, hmm?"

Bob doesn't answer me. I'm not even sure he's heard me. His gaze alternates between the menu and casting about the restaurant, like he's awaiting someone—someone very important. When I'd contacted George to suggest this lunch, I'd told him that, based on my first meeting, I couldn't see much wrong with Bob, that he was lively and loquacious. But here, now, Bob's a silent husk, and George's habitual smile is in retreat.

I look to George, my eyes saying, *Got any ideas about how to kick-start things?* He obliges. "Eric tells me you've done so much for young Ukrainians. Thank you!"

Bob smiles and nods, but his eyes bounce off us, falling upon a passing waitress. "Uh . . . can I get a cheeseburger?"

"Your waitress will be right with you, sir."

"I'd like to change my order . . . to a Reuben and a beer."

"I'm afraid I'm not your waitress, sir. I'll send her over, right away, sir."

"Bob—" I begin.

"I like rocks," says Bob, completely detached from George and me.

"I do, too," I say.

As Bob fingers the fireplace, tilting his head like that dog in those old RCA commercials, I try to keep the momentum going. "We've got a fair bit of stonework at our home. Front walls, walkways, two fireplaces . . . Come to think of it, I spent more time interviewing potential masons than I did choosing my first eye surgeon. Which may explain why I've got such beautiful masonry and such awful eyesight."

George laughs. Once our waitress has come and gone, he takes another crack at engaging Bob. "What's your favorite part of Ukraine? Kiev? The Crimea, maybe?"

Bob doesn't answer, so I do. "The Opera House. Just up the path from the Battleship Potemkin. Where, my research suggests, my grandfather was a leading instigator."

"Really??" exclaims George. "I didn't know. So he's a Ukrainian patriot!"

"I'm not sure I'd go that far, George. He was a Polish patriot, that's for sure, who happened to be studying in Odessa and who despised Russians."

George smiles. "That's good enough for me!"

"Can I get another pickle?" says Bob to the waitress as she sets down his food and beer. "I really like your pickles here."

The frazzled waitress pauses, drinks in this man, his comment, and embraces the poignancy. "Why, thank you. I'll get you all the pickles you want, dear. Just give me a sec."

The remainder of our lunch is more of the same. I'd hoped the guys might chat in Ukrainian. But even speaking a few words in English seems too much for Bob. So I'm consigned to basically acting as Bob's spokesman, telling George how Bob had visited Ukraine several times over the past few years, taught at a top university, was the State Department's Fulbright scholarship scout, and developed this extensive network of loving, deeply indebted young people. George is moved, grateful that Bob's done so much for his fellow Ukrainians. (George had himself established and generously funded a private family foundation providing, among other services, natural family planning and marriage counseling.)

At least Bob's been smiling, for the most part, his appetite's good, and his mind's clear enough to order not just more pickles but also the best beer in the house—two mugs of it. The Czech suds wash down his big sandwich, and then he sets about polishing off the better part of a healthy slice of cheesecake.

After dropping Bob off back home, I immediately ring George from my car to apologize. I thought George would have a blast, but I left the restaurant feeling I'd probably just depressed him as well as me. "Not at all, Eric. It was a great pleasure meeting Bob. I'm sorry he's having such a rough time. He seems like a very special person."

But I don't allow George's graciousness to let me off the hook. As one of Rosalie's tips is *don't assume you know what your patient's desires/*

*needs/feelings are*, I now get the sense that this "great lunch idea" was the product of just such an assumption. I'd assumed what Bob wanted to do; yet it had more to do with what I wanted to do. Had I taken more time—any time!—to review the notes of my orientation and training, perhaps I would have inquired more perceptively, discovering, say, that, rather than venturing out for another meal, maybe Bob would have wanted me to take him to Lake Brittle so he could swim or to Sky Meadow State Park, where, from that magnificent setting and picturesque vantage point, he could paint his beloved white birch trees, red cardinals, and purple blackberries.

## JULY 24

When I next get Bob on the phone, he's rallied. He's back to form. This time I let him direct the conversation. But he doesn't mention swimming or painting. He wants more food. "I love Wegmans' crab soup! It's the best! It's right next door! Can I get some?"

At the store's fabulous seafood bar, where my wife and I often grab a quick, delicious, inexpensive meal, with Bob perched on a high stool and me recollecting how my frail grandmother never recovered from having fallen from her bed, I spend most of my time fretting that he doesn't tumble to the floor. But he slurps safely.

While driving him back to Kathleen's, he and I talk about his trip to Canada—which tops his Bucket List. "It's my own personal slice of heaven." He's been planning it for months, but few of us think he'll ever get there.

"Thanks!" he says, as he opens the car door and heads toward Kathleen's front door. "Thank you," I say. "I'll call you in a few days." He waves goodbye without turning around.

Over the next few weeks, things really go downhill. Canada's looking less and less real, more and more like a dream, a mirage . . . the "Kanada" one can still make out on the walls at Auschwitz, etched in hope . . . by the likes of Viktor Frankl . . . clinging to the flickering flame of deliverance unto a promised land that so many of their relatives had talked about . . . from The Plains of Abraham to Vancouver. I call, often, but either there's no answer or Bob's uninterested in venturing out. He's asleep most of the time now, Kathleen tells me, as well as listless when awake. Higher and higher doses of morphine are administered, more frequently. He's painting less, interacting less, moving more slowly, tripping more often. "He's pretty much depressed all the time," says Kathleen. Her tone adds, *I am, too.*

Just as the trip to Canada's about to be formally scrubbed, Bob roars back from the brink. I show up the day of the departure, unannounced, toting several bags from my favorite deli-bakery. Kathleen opens the door, Bob a few steps behind her. At the sight of the bulging bags, her face turns to mush. She hugs me. "Look what Eric brought, Dad!"

"Oh, boy!" He makes it a small group hug. A Zimmerman sandwich. Once the squeezing subsides, I step away. "A road trip's not complete without proper provisioning. Have a great trip, Bob. A great swim."

## AUGUST 12–17

Kathleen calls. "Any way you can come by tomorrow? My kids have a soccer game."

"Sure. By the way, how'd the trip go?"

"Really well. Surprisingly well. My dad and Uncle Jack drove up to Ohio, picked up my aunt Betsy, and they made it all the way to the Zimmerman family cabin, on the Canadian shore of Lake Erie." Bob doesn't swim much, however, she tells me. "But he dipped his toes."

"I'm so happy for him. By the way, I've called your dad a few times. No answer."

"Yeah. Ever since getting back, he's been out of it most of the time."

The following day, when I arrive, as Kathleen is gathering soccer balls, cleats, and coolers, she says, "Dad'll probably just sleep. He's downstairs, doped up pretty good." Once she splits with her kids, I head downstairs to check on Bob, first passing through an impressively arrayed home gym, with free weights, punching bags, a life-sized dummy, some expensive-looking machines, and other paraphernalia revealing Kathleen's husband's fondness for inflicting bloody mayhem, pursuant to his successful mixed-martial-arts career. The door to Bob's adjacent apartment is slightly ajar. Seeing him asleep, hearing his soft, even breathing, I return back upstairs, find a comfortable chair, and dive into my current book, *Enslaved by Ducks*.

A couple hours later, I'm startled by a piercing wail. I fly downstairs, fumble for the light switch, and, once I can see my way around, enter Bob's cramped quarters. In addition to the bed, there's a card table, stacked with paintings (most notably, myriad renditions of his beloved birch tree); a dresser, on top of which a bunch of pill bottles are lined up, neatly; and a set of instructions, taped to the wall, governing his medication.

He's under the covers, fitful, writhing, moaning, and babbling, unsure whether to get up, or remain in bed. His hands hack at the air—as if fending off some spectral foe. "Oh, it hurts! Oh, Jesus, Lord, take me! I'm ready!"

I feel useless. Clueless. Nonetheless I ask, "Can I get you anything?" "Some milk, please."

I race back upstairs. By the time I've returned with his milk, he's up, seated in a chair beside the card table, at the foot of his bed. While I relocate some paintings, paint brushes, and bottles of paint, so as to have a clear spot to set down his milk, he stares at one particular watercolor. It's a bright sunflower. "God has such a lovely smile," he says, more to himself than to me, before sweeping away a few strands of thin, disheveled hair. Dressed in pajama bottoms and a T-shirt, he looks really frail and brittle.

Several times Bob tries to rise from the chair, but his thighs can't provide sufficient thrust. Each time he descends to the seat, he groans on impact. With each cycle, each struggle, I feel increasingly inept. My thoughts seesaw back and forth, in slow motion, regarding whether to try and help and, if so, how. I feel that I should, but, for some reason, I don't. Something's holding me back, confining me to a mezzanine of observation, willing him to fend for himself. Finally, he manages to rise, almost locking his knees. But then, like an Olympic weightlifter unable to sustain a clean and jerk, Bob collapses, howling as his cancer-pocked bones crumple into the chair. "Oh, Lord! Take me, Lord!"

Now I move toward him, but he stops me, shooting out a hand. Maybe he'd have accepted my help at first, but now it's a matter of pride. He inhales, then clutches the bed sheets for support and balance. But then he releases the sheets and studies his hand, a sad look on his face. I notice the urine-stained sheets. He slumps back into his chair. "Oh," he moans. "Oh . . ." I try not to bite my lip. "Forget about that," I say. "It's nothing."

Upstairs, the front door slams shut, the tremor rattling the pill bottles atop the dresser. A minute later, Kathleen's with us. She immediately takes it all in, strokes Bob's face, and strips the soiled sheets. "Thank you so much," she says to me. "I've got it under control now."

"Sure?" I ask, as Bob sits silently. She nods while balling up the sheets, then hustles into the adjacent laundry room.

That evening, I prepare my report, which includes the following:

Precipitous decline in condition over past 3½ weeks.
(Daughter well aware.) Pain, crying, incoherent.

Later in the evening, Rosalie calls me, informing me that Bob's been rushed to Haymarket Hospice's lone in-patient facility to occupy one of the twenty beds that serve upwards of fifteen hundred patients. The implication is crystal clear: Bob is not expected to last long. Maybe a day or two. Maybe an hour or two.

Yet he's still hanging on when I pop by the Swain Memorial Inpatient Center the next morning. However, he looks totally out of it. His eyes are shut. He looks peaceful, at least.

His younger brother's sitting in a chair, facing Bob. Jack and I have never met or spoken to one another. As I enter, Jack shoots up, smiles, extends his hand, introduces himself, and thanks me—in double time. In his mid-sixties, hair short, shirt polo, khakis pressed, tread on his running shoes well worn, Jack looks fit, clean-cut, and military issue, but he also exudes an easygoing bonhomie. But easygoing oughtn't be confused with easily deterred, as I know from Bob and an Air Force recruiter once learned when he told Jack his eyesight was too weak to be an Air Force pilot. Jack had replied, "Fine. Then watch me be a Navy aviator." The recruiter caved. He knew the Right Stuff when he saw it, even if the eye chart had missed it.

After Jack's given me the sitrep regarding his brother, and just as he starts telling me about his own transition from the Air Force Academy to flying night missions in Laos in 1965, Jack and I are asked to participate in a hastily arranged meeting, joining Bob's daughters, a doctor, a nurse, and the Haymarket Hospice chaplain.

I touch Jack on the elbow, and whisper, "Sure you want me along?"

"Absolutely," he says. "Bob would want you there."

The room is furnished with sofas, easy chairs, drapes, unostentatious rugs, and a piano. It's quiet and tense until the ecumenical caregiver arrives, whereupon, in a soothing tone devoid of judgment, he eases into the dilemma. "We're here to discuss Bob's final wishes, insofar as his funeral arrangements, burial, et cetera. I'm told there's some dis— Ahem. I'm told that Bob's wishes are not crystal clear. Before opening it up for discussion, I'd just like to say two things. First, this sort of thing happens quite often. Second, I'm here only as a moderator, to try and help you, the family, effect Bob's—and your—will."

"I talked a lot about this with Dad," says Jenny, her tone not at all strident. "As you know, he attends River Church a fair bit."

"I also know he's still Catholic," says Kathleen.

That's all that's said for several minutes.

I'm certainly not about to add my two cents. I don't have two cents. Bob's and my spiritual-religious talks have been vague and mystical, such as how, in Bob's opinion, a sunflower is not merely a physical manifestation of botany but a metaphysical expression of an "Ineffable Holy Mystery." Moreover, I've not been asked my opinion, which means, were I to speak, I'd be violating at least three of Rosalie's caregiving guidelines, by: (1) not maintaining proper boundaries (religion topping the list), (2) judging (Rosalie specifically said, *"Don't try to referee family squabbles!"*), and (3) offering unsolicited advice (the fact that I was invited to attend isn't the same as being asked my opinion).

Thankfully, after exchanging some peaceable words, the Zimmerman sisters agree to table the matter. The meeting adjourns, and everyone goes their separate ways.

Jack and I head back into his brother's room, where I pull up beside Bob's pillow. His eyes are still locked tight. I'm not sure what to say. The few thoughts that bubble up inside my head all seem so lame. All I manage is, "You hang in there. Okay?"

He doesn't seem to hear me, but I'm not sure. Not so much as a tiny tic jostles his sheets.

The next day, toward the end of another visit, having left Bob's room, from the hallway I overhear Jack tell his brother, "I love you, Bob."

I pause, struggling against my upbringing. Though very loving, the family forged and spawned by the marriage of Thaddeus Alphonse Lindner to Mary Jean Wellford has never been much for saying *I love you*. My wife and her family changed all this. Her feisty clan having emancipated my emotions, I return to Bob's room.

"Oh, hey," says Jack. "Forget something?"

"Yes."

I pull up close. Bob's eyes are still glued shut. It's hard to tell if he's even breathing. Leaning in close, I whisper, "I love you."

Bob's body convulses in micro-spasms. Though his eyes remain shut, his arm shoots out, and grabs my bicep. "Thank you," he whispers back.

I stare down at his hand. My knees feel like they're about to buckle. But the instant Bob releases his grip, Jack's there to brace me, with an outstretched hand. "Man!" he exclaims. "Those are the first words Bob's said to anyone! On his way up to Canada he talked about you all the time. You've come to mean so much to my brother."

"I can't mean anywhere nears much to Bob . . ." I study Bob's face for a moment, but he appears to have drifted off. "As Bob means to me. And you're the one who's kept your brother going. All these years. Tough years. Plus getting up to the lake and back? What a great gift to give! Bob's slice of heaven."

I return the next day with my wife and daughter in tow. I'd normally not bring either of them. I think like many couples my wife and I orbit in semi-autonomous galaxies. (Among other things, like being a great mother to our two kids, Ellen has her art gallery, tennis, and therapeutic riding volunteer work with autistic children.) But the three of us have just been to Washington, visiting the National Gallery of Art, and are passing right by Bob. I'd hate to miss seeing him, especially if this is going to be his last day on earth.

"You guys don't have to come in," I say, as we're pulling into the parking lot. "I've not told anyone I'd be by today, and I've certainly not suggested you might. Plus, I know this is a bit odd, as you've never met Bob or any of his family."

"No," says Ellen. "I'd like to, seeing how you've described him and his family." My wife looks to Sarah, who says, "I'm good. Sure, why not? If you think they're okay with us just showing up, out of the blue."

"I know they'll be okay with it," I say. "More than okay."

Once inside, we find Bob still hanging on, his eyes still shut, his breathing much more labored. After a few moments, Jack walks in and flashes his big smile. "Hello!" he says. "I'm Jack Zimmerman, Bob's younger brother. Let me guess—you must be Ellen, and you must be Sarah." They both nod, and they all shake hands. "Eric talks about you all the time."

Ellen eyes me for a second, wondering if Jack is talking hooey, but then he says, "You two are the tennis hotshots, right? The all-star mother-daughter team from Warrenton?" "Hardly," says Ellen, "but it's nice he described us that way!"

*Thanks, Jack!* I say with a smile.

"My girls are runners," says Jack.

"Talk about all-stars," I say.

We chitchat a bit more; then, after his cell phone rings, Jack steps outside, into the hallway. This gives Sarah occasion to step closer and have a better look at Bob. She's a lot like Bob in that her default setting is to smile and remain upbeat. It takes a lot to overcome her temperament. Here it's overcome. Her face is very expressive, and it's now expressing great sadness, as well as an appreciation for how lucky she is to be so young and so healthy.

I return the next day to find the ever-faithful Jack. I've interrupted his cat nap, but he yawns, stretches, and snaps to attention. He briefs me, concluding with, "Basically, no change. Bob's not opened his eyes for days and not said a word, either. The docs say he probably won't do either, ever again."

"I'm so sorry, Jack. I'll miss . . . those eyes of his."

"Me—" Jack's voice catches. His face flushes; his eyes glimmer with pretears. "Yep."

From the bedside table, I lift the frame that contains a photo of Bob, from his trip to Canada. He's seated in an Adirondack chair, outside his boyhood cabin, beside his beloved lake. Wrapped in an orange-and-black checkered shawl, he's surrounded by loved ones, smiling inscrutably. I try making small talk, which is always hazardous for me. "Any traveling on the horizon, Jack?"

"Playing it by ear," he responds charitably to my numbskull question. "You?"

I tell him my wife and I are heading up to see an exhibition on the Dead Sea Scrolls. "Heading . . . up? Where to?"

"Canada."

Bob stirs. Jack and I both start, as if shocked by a low-voltage charge. "Hea . . ." Bob mutters.

And then he's gone.

Jack and I stare at one another. We're not sure if Bob's final word was going to be *heaven*, but we are sure that's where he's headed.

## AUGUST 26

En route to the memorial service in Winchester at River Church, while driving past Sky Meadows State Park, one of my favorite places to hike with Ellen, I'm feeling pretty good about my first assignment—until this patting myself on the back strikes me as prideful and even a bit morbid. But it's fair to assume, I think, at least, that a dying patient longed for companionship and, at least according to Rosalie, Jack, Kathleen, and Jenny, I helped out.

Yet . . . as I watch the diverse crowd stream into Jenny's strip-mall outlet of spirituality, laughing, crying, and chatting in several languages, a query bubbles to the surface, threatening to pop my assumption: Why'd Bob need *me*? The place is already jammed, and I know that loads more would be here, too, if they'd had more notice, or weren't in Kiev or Manila, Hanoi or Bangkok. Jack's told me that once word got around that Bob was in hospice, the outpouring of love and concern was overwhelming. E-mails, texts, and phone calls poured in by the hundreds.

I love the sermon by Jenny's husband, Mark. It's muscular, in keeping with this big, tall ball of evangelical energy who finds it not only impossible but also just plain wrong not to shout from the rooftops the Good News that saved him from Gehenna. After the service, Mark and I share a laugh over this Russian Orthodox family we both knew growing up and how the matriarch used to give him hell for taking the Lord's name in vain. "That Mrs. Gambal sure laid into me!" he says.

Driving home, my caregiving veers into more personal territory. I ring my folks down in Boynton Beach, Florida, where they spend most of the year. "Hey, Dad," I say, to my eighty-three-year-old father, "how are things with you and Mom?" (She's also eighty-three.)

"We're better now."

"Now?"

"I mean we're back from the hospital."

"The hospital?? I didn't know!"

"Oh," he says. My folks sometimes forget whom they've told what, expecting that if one of their four kids is told something it'll be relayed along the family grapevine. In this case it's not been.

"Who went?" I ask.

"We both did. Your mother and I."

"I mean . . . who needed to go? Why? What's going on? Everything's okay now, though?"

"Your mother . . . She . . . It was nothing."

"What was 'nothing,' Dad?"

Some klutzy muffled sounds tell me my ex-CIA mom has just picked up, on the other line. Her eavesdropping tradecraft is a bit rusty, exacerbated by her being half-deaf.

I play dumb to the existence of the party line. "She okay now?"

"I think so."

"But I still don't—"

"Darn it!" curses my not-so-clandestine mom, after dropping the phone.

"What'd the doc say, Dad?" Assumption one: "How long did it take for the ambulance to get to Pine Tree?"

"Umm . . ."

"Dad?"

"Tad!" Mom whispers, snappishly.

"What??" he fires back. "Umm, we didn't take an ambulance."

Assumption two: "How long did it take for the cab to arrive, then?"

"Umm . . ."

"Tad!"

"Dad?"

"We didn't take a cab, Eric. We waited an awfully long time! So, finally, I drove—"

"You drove??"

"Umm . . ."

"But, Dad! You're *blind*!"

"Not entirely. Plus, I didn't need to see. I know the way. I took nothing but right turns."

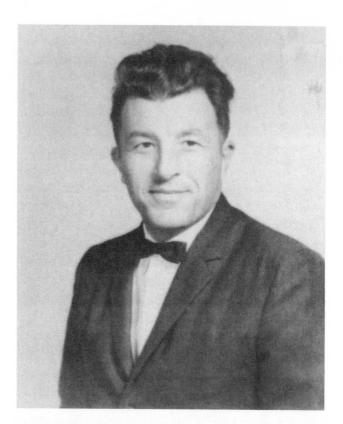

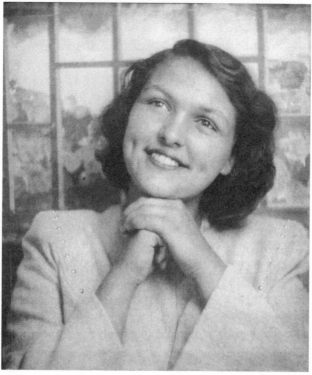

# ADVERSITY CRUMBLES
# WHEN LAUGHED AT

**M**y mostly blind dad ignoring me about getting behind the wheel of a car immediately after my first patient, half-blind, teaches me a thing or two about the expanded vision his blindness occasioned gets me wondering what else I'm not seeing, what other of Rosalie Palermo's *Dos* and *Don't*s I must be violating. *Don't take on more patients than you can manage . . .* Is my volunteer caregiving crowding out or otherwise jeopardizing my "family caregiving," seeing as my parents are both ten years older than Bob? *Do listen to your patients . . .* I'm hearing my parents, for the most part, but am I really listening to what it is they're trying to say?

Two things, at least, are clear. First, I've ignored this tip: *Don't expect your patient to conform to your standards or expectations . . .* by erroneously assuming that my dad would behave as I wanted him to. Second, the "team" handling my parents' care is not communicating well. *Do communicate with your fellow caregivers . . .*

Though my three siblings and I all live in the D.C. area and get along fine, we seldom communicate, let alone coordinate. But with my blind eighty-three-year-old dad driving my deaf eighty-three-year-old mom around Florida's NASCAR track, my two older brothers, younger sister, and I realize things have gotten a bit out of hand and that the key to helping our folks starts with us—committing to communicating better, and more openly, through the loud clutter of our largely disconnected lives, not unlike how the Zimmerman daughters were compelled to engage in dialogue at the in-patient center, pertaining to their father's funeral preferences. My siblings and I meet for lunch in Georgetown. The first thing we do is agree that we've got to do a better job of staying in touch. Then we agree that, somehow, we've got to convince our folks to move from their Florida villa into assisted-living accommodations, and persuade them that ceding some independence doesn't imply any ceding of pride.

It won't be easy. My folks are proud. They've done very well for themselves—on their own. They prize their independence and solitude. They're used to—and prefer—helping others, not vice versa.

We've got to get Thaddeus Alphonse to stop thinking he's James Bond, his Ford Taurus an Aston Martin. We don't think Dad will fight us much about giving up driving—just golfing, seeing as he hates driving a cart ("They ruined the game"), preferring to walk. For more than twenty years, an enjoyable ten-minute walk put him on the tee at a primo golf course. I've known few people in my life as passionate about anything as my dad is about golf.

But Dad's not the main hurdle, nor is golf his primary passion. Mom is. And so everything about Operation Sunset must be clandestine until my siblings and I get all our ducks in a row. Moreover, even assuming we *can* get them in a row, unless Mom thinks the idea of moving is entirely hers, it'll never stand a chance.

Ann, Gary, Rusty, and I draw straws. Mine's the shortest, so I'm pressed into service.

Under the guise of a routine visit by a caring son, I pack for Florida. My mission: covertly find a suitable new home for my folks and report back to my siblings.

Agent Wellford is ready for me. Not for nothing was Mary Jean Wellford one of the first women hired by Allen Dulles, the CIA's legendary spymaster. While Mom always says her job "really wasn't that interesting," she also says she took an oath never to reveal what she did. So, her being a spook, trained in disinformation, etc., it didn't shock me (as a ten-year-old) to stumble across a hidden cache of pocket (or purse) language booklets one day (Turkish, Farsi, Arabic) in our Maryland home (safe house), as if they'd fallen out of Mom's tattered go kit. Not only did it not shock me, it thrilled me. Suddenly everyone else's mom was so boring. Other kids' moms ran with the Girl Scouts, selling cookies, while my mom ran with the OSS studs who'd parachuted behind enemy lines, inspiring Ian Fleming's tales of derring-do. Suddenly it all made sense: why my natural-born, speed-reading mom devoured every book that hit the shelves pertaining to espionage or the Cold War; why, when my folks had neighbors over, Mom was always off huddled in a corner, chatting with an IBM exec whose globetrotting led everyone to suspect he was a CIA asset (which was confirmed forty years later); why, while everyone else was yakking, Mom was often situated in the corner, just observing, listening, surveilling, like that scarily inscrutable femme fatale with the knitting needles in *A Tale of Two Cities*.

Once my boots are on the ground in the Sunshine State, Operation Sunset appears to be proceeding according to plan. At least I *think* I'm having some success maneuvering Mom into, first, liking the idea of moving to a place with better access to medical care while also dispensing with certain drudgeries (e.g., pruning fecund palm trees, exterminating dachshund-size roaches) and, second, believing that the move is her idea.

## OCTOBER 21, 2009

Rosalie e-mails me. I call her. She briefs me. I agree to add another lady in her eighties to my caregiving roster, but, apparently, there are some strings attached. "Your official patient is Ellen Hensley, but I've signed you up for the family plan!"

Ellen, seventy-nine, has advanced-stage Alzheimer's, and, while she's the only official patient, apparently the Hensley household resembles a small hospital ward. Her eighty-eight-year-old diabetic husband, Elmer, suffers from a weak heart and acute arthritis. And though she's the primary caregiver, their fifty-six-year-old daughter, Barbara, is also quite ill. Their only other child, Lake, fifty-eight, lives two hours south, in Harrisonburg, where he's the maintenance supervisor for one of the world's largest turkey producers. Lake and his wife, Pam, have given Ellen and Elmer their only grandchild, David, who, like Lake, is big into Civil War history and reenactments.

Ellen was born in Mount Hope, West Virginia, which I've driven though a few times and know as a place where King Coal vies with Saint Paul, where billboards proclaiming, "Coal—it keeps the lights on!" battle others citing Colossians, Philippians, and Romans. It's a place you don't want to be driving through during snow or ice storms, what with all the twisting and turning up and around the jagged, clear-cut mountains. It's a place that, despite all the rocks, rattlesnakes, and righteousness, produces the nicest people I've ever met. It's a place where the state slogans make sense: the first was "Wild and Wonderful"; then, after John Denver's mega hit, the Mountaineer legislators in Charleston added "Almost Heaven." In my experience, West Virginians are wild and wonderful and heaven isn't a figment of their collective imagination. They believe in fire and brimstone but can also husband all manner of tasty, high-proof produce in a few millimeters of the stony soil that, to the less industrious, seems unforgiving.

Ellen left Mount Hope to get her teaching certificate at Radford University, just across the state line, into the Virginia that West Virginia hived itself from in 1863. Afterward, she headed 150 miles north, where she taught for the next thirty-six years in the largest of the D.C. area's surrounding seventeen counties, Fairfax, home to more than one million. Early in her career, she met a young Marine from Haymarket, Virginia, just back from California.

Their meeting in Virginia had been a fluke. Elmer was supposed to be in Korea, fighting the Commies. But, just after enlisting, while at Boot Camp, his appendix burst—nearly killing him. So, after the Corps said, "Thanks, but no thanks," Elmer packed up his duffel bag and returned East. He didn't know what to do with his Piedmont skill set. Prior to enlisting in the Marines, he'd trapped game, earning $1 for mink pelts and 25¢ for skunk, which then were fashioned into fancy coats for the Great Gatsby types. He shot deer, rabbit, and squirrel to put food in his belly. And then—personally—he shot down hundreds of Japanese planes while serving in the Coast Guard during World War II. After several false starts, he ended up applying his terrific hand-eye coordination to the butchering trade and ended up working at Safeway for more than thirty years.

"They're devout Christians," adds Rosalie. "All three of them. Ellen and Elmer, I'm told, used to love crisscrossing the country by car, often stopping to dig for rocks. Elmer had an amazing rock collection, much of which he lost in a fire. I know Ellen at least used to play the piano, but I'm not sure she does much playing these days. Finally, Elmer loves doing all sorts of stuff outdoors—gardening, farming, chopping wood."

"And the daughter?" I ask. "Is she employed?"

"I'm not sure," says Rosalie. "She's listed as the primary caregiver, though in addition to periodic visits from the Haymarket Hospice nurse they've arranged for private nursing care . . . Here, let me see . . ." I hear some papers rattling. "Nurses are there Monday through Friday, from one P.M. to seven thirty P.M."

"So, the best time for me is weekdays, before one, and weekends?"

"Right."

"You say Barbara's the 'primary caregiver.' Is she a nurse?"

"I don't think so. But she does sound quite intelligent, and pleasant. But . . ."

"Yes?"

"I'm told she's morbidly obese."

"I've never really understood what that meant."

"I know. It's a vague term. It essentially means that her weight is so excessive it brings with it a host of very serious collateral health issues."

"It all sounds so very sad." My mind drifts to Bob's lesson on empathy. "And . . . it takes me back. I was certainly very obese as a teenager. It's no fun."

"I find that very hard to believe."

"Well, it's true. Back then I was eleven inches shorter, forty-seven pounds heavier, with a stratospheric BMI."

"You'd never guess it, today." Rosalie clears her throat. "One more thing. I need to warn you . . . Our social worker, Lee Lund, tells me the house is . . . well . . . really messy."

## OCTOBER 29

I pull into the driveway of a modest rambler, behind an old Olds that (I'd wager) hasn't passed state inspection in quite some time. Beside me is a more recent vintage Chevy coupe, parked behind a later-model Honda. Between the cars and the backyard is a hand-cranked International Harvester tractor, spilling out from under a rusted, splay-legged carport. In the middle of the backyard are two trailers, one hitched to a truck, beside a log splitter, a massive tree stump, mounds of bricks and wood (covered with plastic tarp), and a small, red Radio Flyer wagon, brimming with firewood. Off a ways, beyond a small pond, a decrepit mobile camper buckles amid a dense tangle of dogwood, ivy, and weeds.

I pull into a parallel patch of gravel, grass, and oil stains, step from my car, and walk toward the front door. Vines heavy with mature yellow tomatoes and ripening green peppers pack the twelve-inch strip of topsoil between the concrete walkway and the rambler's brick foundation. On the stoop, a ceramic owl begins hooting the moment I start rapping on the ornately carved door.

"Come on in!" a woman cries out, drowning out the owl.

I push open the heavy door and enter an obstacle course. I sidestep spiraled piles of books, magazines, and newspapers and wend my way around whittled tree limbs, random rock piles, bags of bagels, and tubes of potato chips. Against the wall, on an upright piano's bench, half-drunk two-liter bottles of Coke and Mountain Dew fizz like carbonated sentinels with a taste for sonatas.

"In here!" cries the same female voice, somewhere beyond the soft drinks.

I make my way into the kitchen, past a long table covered with papers, unopened mail, and Tupperware containers full of keys, change, hearing-aid batteries, and whatnot. An armada of dishes, pots, and pans floats about in the sink. Yet . . . a lovely aroma slices through the clutter: a wood fire.

I arrive in the den. Small to begin with, the room contains a big fireplace, surrounded by floor-to-ceiling logs, two sofas, one La-Z-Boy recliner, various tables, a TV mounted within a bookcase—from which Drew Carey addresses a game-show contestant—and five people, three of whom are quite large. I pause, smile, and wave.

"Hi!" says Ellen and Elmer's elder child, from one of the sofas. "I'm Barbara." She's big; I guess as heavy as the All-Pro Redskins lineman who used to live near me, but a lot shorter. However, in her loose blouse and flip-flops, with her ruddy, smiling face and strong, spirited voice, she seems, if not the picture of health, hardly "morbid." She studies me while nudging the glasses up the bridge of her nose, then reciprocates my smile.

Everyone seems amused, in fact. Her, her parents (so I presume), and the dark-skinned nurse, a third of Barbara's size. It's as if they hadn't expected me to navigate through their version of the corn mazes that dot this part of Virginia during fall harvest time or make it through the kitchen without tripping over a sack of potatoes.

What am I missing? Rosalie's briefing led me to expect profound sadness. Yet all I see and sense is unbridled cheerfulness.

Barbara addresses my patient. "Momma, this is Eric Lindner. He's with hospice. He's gonna spend some time with you to help out Daddy and me."

From her recliner, Ellen gives me the up-down. She's a large woman, too (though nowhere near as big as Barbara). Her mostly white hair, which retains some streaks of auburn, doesn't quite reach to her shoulder. She's wearing glasses and a floral nightgown. Her twin dimples—her signal feature—are lovely. "Very well, then. Don't just stand there. Find a desk, take a seat, and join the rest of the class."

There are no desks. This is no classroom. Or so I think.

I glance at my supposed caregiving ally, the small-boned, big-eyed, coffee-skinned nurse. But she's no help, staring at me, blankly, like a cuddly Sri Lankan lemur.

I turn to Barbara. She shrugs. Her eyes say, *Get used to it*. "Shakespeare said 'All the world's a stage.' Well, for Momma? All the world's a classroom."

I pivot to Elmer, a solidly built man with a thick head of white hair, who radiates a loopy brio. The first words out his mouth are "Caught me a rabbit today! Critter feasting on my turnips!" His forceful thigh slap suggests he's not angry at the rabbit, just happy he's bested him. "Like turnips, don't you?" Before I can answer him, he throws his head back and howls.

"Turnips?" I stare at the nurse.

She stares back, then covers her sparkling teeth with a hand to suppress a giggle.

"Daddy grows the best turnips!" exclaims Barbara.

Elmer's cement-truck shoulders shake, rattling and animating the talking trout on the mantle, which cries out, "Throw me back! Throw me back!"

Ellen's ignoring Elmer, something I guess she's perfected over six decades of marriage. I offer her my hand. "Nice to meet you," I say. Turning away from Drew Carey (who's in the process of signing off), she takes my hand, and we shake. "Well now," she says, "nice to meet you."

I love Ellen's thick coal-country drawl, which reminds me of this sweet West Virginia redhead I once fancied. As Ellen smiles—which seems as natural to her as breathing is to me—her dimples pucker. This cues another round of smiling: husband, daughter, nurse—and me.

"Got me some delicious turnips!" Elmer reminds me. "And gonna have me a delicious rabbit stew, too! Circle of life! Hah!"

The nurse looks away, covering her mouth again to stifle another bout of giggling.

The trout tapers off: "Throw me back! Throw . . . me . . . ."

"Well," I say, "not sure I've ever eaten a turnip, Elmer. May I call you Elmer?"

"'*Course*! What else'd you call me!? *Hah!*"

"Well, Elmer, probably never having eaten one, I can't say whether I'd like a turnip or not. But I'm game to try one of yours."

"Biggest ones you'll ever lay your eyes on! Just volunteered to grow, up out in my backyard. Rabbits and squirrels get lots of 'em. Dig under the fence. Least I keep the deer out, and the foxes. I eat the turnips raw. Love 'em!"

Ignoring her husband's turnip treatise, Ellen asks of me, "You do your homework?"

Before I can respond, a famous tune yanks everyone's attention toward the TV screen. The *Bonanza* theme song: Bum-dada bum-dada bum-dada bum-dada Da-Daaaaa . . .

Ellen switches from pedagogy to The Ponderosa: "*Bonanza*! Hoss! He's so cute!"

"Little Joe's my favorite," says Barbara.

"Veddy hun-some," says the Sri Lankan cowgirl, nodding. "Veddy sweet."

"Ever heard of the Grey Ghost?" the Hoss-like Elmer asks me, abruptly changing his channel from reruns and turnips to Civil War insurgents.

"Yep," I say. "Colonel John Singleton Mosby, the dashing guerilla commander during the Civil War. Or, as my mother—her people are from Tidewater Virginia—still prefer, the War of Northern Aggression."

"Exactly!" says Barbara.

"I caught me my rabbit, but ole Abe never caught the Grey Ghost!"

Ellen's attention remains fixed on the tube. For most of this initial visit, she ignores me. She seems tired and, perhaps, shy; watching TV is less awkward, less of a drain. "Look!" she blurts, referring to a cat food commercial. "What a cute kitty." Then she shifts gears, in reverse. Fifty years in reverse. "Barb, dear? Now don't you forget your lunch. There's a nice peach in there for you."

My report of this first visit includes this excerpt:

Patient delightful. Quiet. Stationary. Didn't once move from her recliner, during two-hour visit. Appears to be living more in her "Alzheimer's world" than the "real world."

But, though still a rookie caregiver, one thing I understand is the mercurial nature of my patients, as reflected in my second report, submitted just two days later:

Patient still delightful. Still insisting she's a teacher, as she was decades ago. But, today, patient not so quiet and not at all stationary. She's manic. Constantly, abruptly, up and about. To play the piano and/or "head off to school."

## NOVEMBER 9

I arrive to find Elmer, Barbara, and a nurse sprawled about, fast asleep. Ellen's hoisting herself off the floor.

I rush over to her, reaching for her. "You okay??"

"Just a small spill. Why hello, Eric!" She's chipper. She seems completely with it.

I've read that the concussive effect of even simply bumping into the corner of a table can snap an Alzheimer's patient back into temporary lucidity, which I assume is what's going on here.

Unfortunately, subsequent visits confirm my assumption. Though certain faculties are more resistant than others, the disease's memory-wiping feature marches on, erasing many of Ellen's most basic recollections. Such as, How do I move from point A to point B? Why are people placing stuff in front of me and telling me to eat? What purpose does it serve, putting whatever this is in my mouth? What did you say this is called? A fork? It does what? One Alzheimer's symptom is the cutting off of communication between the stomach and the brain. Or, when one side of the brain is talking, the receiving end hears only gibberish. Every now and then the dramatic falloff in Ellen's calorie intake shuts down her breathing or weakens her so that she collapses. Then 911's dialed, the Lake Jackson Rescue Squad arrives, and Ellen's rushed to the ER.

Back at the Hensky home one day, her mother and father asleep, Barbara tells me how her mom's recently been running a combination marathon–obstacle course, alternating between peaceful, sonorous rest and sudden, frenetic running about. Rushing toward her piano to flip through some sheet music and bang out a stanza or two, springing over to the bookcase to rummage around for her school lesson plans, snatching the car keys and making a break for the front door to head off to her imaginary school. "We're exhausted!" says Barbara.

"Indeed we are," adds Elmer from the sofa, opening his eyes. "She's plum tuckered us out. Hah! That's my girl!"

Most of the time, however, Ellen's fast asleep, which means most of the companionship I'm providing is for Elmer and/or Barbara, and vice versa. Though eclectic, most of the Hensley curriculum revolves around Jesus Christ and Barack Obama.

"I'm telling you," says Barbara, "he's the Antichrist!"

"As slippery as any snake I've ever seen," adds Elmer, his smile and laugh suggesting he likes snakes.

"'Course," continues Barbara, "if he is the Antichrist, then the Rapture's just around the corner, and I've got me a first-class ticket! So, in the grand scheme of things, who cares??"

"Amen, baby girl! Amen!"

Though bored by the political part of the syllabus, Scripture resurrects Ellen. "Tempteth not the Lord!" says Ellen, awakening.

"Sorry, Momma."

"'Let no man,'" Ellen continues, "'say when he is tempted; I am tempted of God: for God cannot be tempted with evil, neither tempteth he any man!'"

"James one, thirteen," says Barbara, looking at me.

"A—men!" says Elmer.

Barbara's sin forgiven, Ellen turns to me, her smile stretching her dimples. "I especially liked that coconut ice cream you brought me last time. Yum!"

"I'm glad," I respond, even though I've never brought her coconut. Last time I brought her Rocky Road, strawberry, and chocolate mint chip. She ate a scoop of each. Or, being more precise, dripped and plopped as much onto her dressing gown as she spooned into her mouth. "I'll have to bring you more, then. Is coconut your favorite flavor?"

But by now she's nodded off again, snoring like a tugboat.


## NOVEMBER 13

I arrive to another episode of *Bonanza*. While pointing at Dan Blocker's nineteenth-century Western duds, Ellen cries out, "I really liked Drew's suit today!" Then she hauls herself out of her chair, makes good time padding across the room, and stops, staring at a framed photo, on a shelf. "We weren't courting yet . . . but doesn't Elmer look mighty handsome in his Marine getup? Boy, do I love a man in uniform!" Then she nods at me: "You ever wear a uniform?"

Before I can answer, she's back to her chair and on the Ponderosa. "Such pretty horses!"

The rest of my visit is just as manic, but not as much fun . . .

Patient very agitated today. Constantly up and down between chair and
wheelchair. Moaning. Sad. Daughter very upset. Met Haymarket Hospice
nurse, husband's physical therapist.


## NOVEMBER 20

Where I live, the cell phone reception can be very spotty. So it's not
until I get up and over the mountain and into town that I see Barbara's
been trying to get ahold of me. Frantically.

"Momma's been rushed to the hospital," she tells me once I ring her.

"Prince William?"

"Yes," says Barbara, crying.

"I'll get there as soon as I can."

When I arrive, I see no one anywhere in the vicinity of Ellen's room.
My mind shoots back to that scene in the *Godfather* when Michael
shows up, expecting to see a crowd, but he's all alone.

It's not long before people start streaming in, however. For the first
time, I meet Barbara's brother, Lake; his wife, Pam; and some friends
of the family. They all seem very nice and—surprisingly—relaxed. At
peace.

All except Lake's sister, that is. She's in bits, slumped in a chair in the
hallway. Ellen's been such a great companion for her, especially since
the collapse of her marriage. The apparent, imminent likelihood of no
longer having her mom around is very hard for Barbara. Normally loquacious, she doesn't say a word.

Elmer seems serene, relaxed, ebullient. I know why, too, for while
visiting his mostly sleeping wife or while Ellen's been fixated on the
TV, Elmer and I have had occasion to spend hours together. So I know
Elmer to be both a staunch Christian, certain that his wife's "going to a
better place," and a fierce fighter who understands that to fight ably one
must stay serene, relaxed, ebullient.

I sense that Ellen's been his softening agent. Elmer never smiles in
the old photos around the house. In them he looks fierce. Like he could

take out a tank with his bare hands. In them I can see how he shot down—himself—dozens of Japanese planes a day.

"A day??" I'd said.

"Yessir. We average a hundred and fifteen a day. The entire ship, I mean."

"Averaged??"

"Yessir. Still got me the ship's log."

Caring for Ellen is Elmer's toughest battle—by far. Tougher than his grueling, terrifying stints at Iwo Jima and Okinawa. "The Zeros come at us like great swarms of hornets, seventy-five at a time." Tougher than his short-lived tour with the Marines. Tougher than losing his beloved home to a fire and having to rebuild from scratch. Tougher than battling with the insurance lawyers who denied coverage or un-Christian-sounding Christian lawyers who gypped him out of a big gift. Tougher than trying to comfort his big baby girl, Barbara, who, upon learning that her husband was gay, leading a double-life, just about gave up on her own life, quitting work, eating herself into oblivion.

Now he's fighting for Ellen. But this man who can skin a skunk without getting stinky and shoot down a Zero from four miles away—is now at a loss. For whom, how, and what do you fight when your foe is Alzheimer's?

## NOVEMBER 24

Arrived in morning, just before patient returned home from hospital. Family a wreck. Exhausted. Sad. Confused.

The doctors don't give the Hensleys much to go on, either in terms of a diagnosis or a prognosis. Alzheimer's is very capricious.

Most days Ellen's asleep much of the day and night. When up, she's very weak.

But Ellen's a fighter, too. One minute, she's snoring soundly in her recliner—then springs up, bolts over to the piano, takes a seat, and starts flipping through sheet music.

"Momma!" yells Barbara. "Use your walker!"

"What is it, dear?" says Elmer, rubbing the sleep from his eyes.

"Mrs. Hensley!" pleads one Sri Lankan, in her sing-song English.

"Please," says another Sri Lankan, brought in as reinforcement.

During such episodes, for the most part, I just sit and watch. Not having a clue what to do or say. In fact, I often wonder what value I could possibly be providing. I've no medical training, I don't know CPR, and I couldn't even do a Heimlich maneuver were there a gun to my head. They've got a nurse 24/7. (Often, two overlap for an hour or so.) A doctor's on call. The highly responsive, friendly Lake Jackson EMS crew is right around the corner. What's more, I've not attended church in a decade (apart from a few funerals), and most of what this family likes to talk about has to do with Scripture, in one fashion or another. My BBA, MBA, and JD seem odd "qualifications," indeed.

Ellen's seated at the piano, tinkling the ivories. "I've got to get to school!"

"School's out, dear," says Elmer, from the sofa. "Don't need to go no more. You've done your part. Time for you to rest."

Ellen spins round on the piano bench, growls, and barks, "NO! I've got to go! Who'll teach the children??" Then she swivels back around and begins playing a lovely etude.

It's very hard watching Ellen suffer, to observe her dutifulness, her frustration, her inability to do what her slipping mind has convinced her she must do.

In fact, it seems easier for Elmer than it does for me. He looks at me and smiles, as if he can read my mind and would like to clue me in on the paradox. "She taught for twenty-six years. She was committed, and she was tough. She didn't give out many As."

"When did—"

"It all began about eight years ago . . ."

Ellen's condition has ebbed and flowed ever since. Once the ebbs started to overwhelm the flows, it was time to make the hard decision so many have to make: Refuse to surrender hope and seek a miraculous cure? Or focus on caring, not curing? On the quality of life, as opposed to a quantitative extension?

The Hensley family believes wholeheartedly in miracles. But they're neither ostriches nor bitter clingers to fundamentalist dogma. They're very smart and extremely well read. They want Ellen to enjoy her remaining days, not struggle.

"Momma knows this life isn't the one that really matters," says Barbara.

Elmer nods. "Amen, baby girl!"

He turns to me. "One night, in the middle of the night, I notice she's not in bed. So I come out to look for her. She's sitting on the floor. Pulled all the books off the shelves. Dumped them onto the floor. When I ask her what she's doing, she tells me, 'Why, silly! Getting ready for school!' But she's saying this twenty years after she'd retired. Now the doctors, they can't tell me what caused it. A few days later, I find a mark on her. A bite of some sort, but unlike any I'd seen a'fore. She got bit by a Brown Recluse spider."

"I remember those," I say. "Never actually seen one. Like a Black Widow?"

"Worse," says Barbara. "But the doctors can't tell if the bite has something to do with her condition or not."

"But it probably didn't help," I say.

Elmer nods. "That's a fact."

Periodic breaks in his fight for Ellen allow Elmer to attend to his other love, apart from his family, and his faith: the outdoors. Elmer is particularly passionate about wood. He seems to know everything there is to know about wood. How best to saw it, split it. What's best for whittling, cooking, heating, making furniture. "Locust makes the best fence posts, white oak the best firewood. Pin oak you can't hardly cut, the grain's so gnarly."

One of the simplest, most appreciated ways I help out is, when he knows I've got Ellen covered, Elmer can head outdoors to work alongside Brother Wood. I know it's about time for me to leave when I see him pull up to the den's sliding glass door, towing his creaky red Radio Flyer wagon, filled with the black walnut he spends so much time splitting, carting, and loading into his fireplace.

Every now and then he'll ask me to help. "Lend me a hand? Hold the wedge? Used to be there wasn't no stump I couldn't lick my own self. But those days are long gone."

The idea of holding a sharp iron wedge so an eighty-nine-year old arthritic ex-Marine can bring down a sledgehammer an inch or so from my hands isn't the most appealing of propositions. But though he wobbles a bit when he walks, his hand-eye coordination seems not to have suffered much, if at all, from his days shooting down kamikazes or cleaving and packaging an Angus steer faster and cleaner than any of Safeway's five thousand other butchers.

Though wood's his specialty, the general range of his outdoor expertise is breathtaking. Such as how to keep the deer from destroying my rose bushes. "Go to the game warden, ask to rub a rag along the inside of the cage they use to transport the dead coyotes brought in for bounty, then, when you get home, wet the rag, and wring it out into your bushes. Your deer problems'll be gone."

Or how to keep the field mice from getting inside my car to eat the gorp I keep there. "Got lots of seeds in it?"

"Yes it does. And nuts and fruits."

"Hoo, boy! That's mice talk for the Country Cookin' all-you-can-eat buffet!"

"Any way to stop 'em?"

"Sure. You using a plastic bag now, I bet, right?"

"Yes."

"Start using an empty peanut butter jar. They can't smell through it or chew through it."

Elmer's outdoor proficiency arose out of necessity. "Back in thirty-six, weren't no jobs anywhere. But I'd get me a dollar for every mink pelt, two bits for skunk. Once, I'm out trying to catch me a mink, see, and the darn thing near rips me to shreds. Pound for pound, nothing's more ferocious than mink, including badgers."

"I didn't even know minks were around here."

"Not as many today as back then. All the development's driven 'em off."

"What happened to that one you caught back in thirty-six?"

His eyes light up, as Homer's must've when he first talked of Troy. "Well, see, I'd cornered her in this hollow [sounds like *holler*] of a big linden branch, high up. But then she pounces and bites onto my arm. Fortunately, I have me on a thick coat."

"Wow! How old were you?"

"Twelve. Maybe thirteen. But I was scrappy. So the mink and I, we both fall out the tree, onto the ground. Darn near broke my neck! But I wriggle out of my coat, wrap the ornery critter up, throw her into the cage, and slam the door. We eat real good that night. Yessir!"

Mostly, however, rather than catch lethal critters with his bare hands, he kills them with great marksmanship. The same skill he'd used to keep his belly full during the Depression he later used to save many an American life at Iwo Jima and Okinawa. "They were sneaky, too. Never know'd where they're coming from or heading to. Sometimes they'd fly solo. Other times they'd come in great clusters.

"After this one cluster attack, later that same night, in the dark, when they usually didn't fly, I catch a glimpse, way off in the distance. Just a flicker, against the moon. It's this larger fighter bomber—not a Zero— flying slow, low. Too low for the radar to pick up.

"I'm worried, 'cause I think it's beyond reach of my forty. So this fella's hugging the coast, camouflaged by the trees, making a beeline for another LST. But . . . I manage to lock him in my sights, and I start a-shootin'."

"You get him, Elmer?"

He smiles humbly. "Caught a break. Got lucky. Hit him just before he reaches the LST. Some shrapnel hits our boys. Some get burned. But no one's kilt."

"Think of all the lives you saved, Elmer! All the children and grand-children born because of your even seeing that plane. Then your shoot-ing it down, from four miles away! And the irony! You survive how many near-death situations in and around Iwo Jima, Okinawa, and elsewhere? Only to nearly die from a burst appendix? In *California*?"

"Ha! My stint with the Marines was sure mighty short! I was lucky! That fighting in Korea wasn't no picnic. I've surely caught my share of blessings!

"Oh!" He remembers something. "Got something for you." He hoists himself up out of his chair and walks to the kitchen table, where he grabs something. He hides it behind his back while returning to me. "Ready for a taste sensation?"

"Sure."

He hands me something that resembles a cross between a pumpkin and an onion.

"A turnip?"

"That's about as good as it gets, when it comes to turnips, if I do say so myself."

That's about as braggy as he gets. He normally says such-and-such "volunteered to grow" or "I caught me some favorable weather." But he's just being humble. The evidence unequivocally points to a very green thumb, including the gargantuan turnip.

Which I eat. Raw. I'm surprised by its slightly sweet, earthy taste. It's crisp, crunchy, and juicy. "This is delicious, Elmer!"

"Came up even better and bigger at the old place."

"That fire must've been really hard."

He shrugs. "I ever tell you about the fella I bought this place from?"

"No."

"Now, he could work with wood! From West Virginia, like my bride. Best gun maker I ever seen."

"Gun maker?" I ask. "People still make guns?"

"In West Virginia? You name it, they make it. Pretty much. Guns. Liquor. Medicine. Clothes. They are, by God, a self-sufficient people. They will be, I reckon, the last holdouts on the Day of Reckoning."

Elmer goes on to tell me how before he bought his current home, while walking through it, he came upon a room where he found 123 shotguns and rifles. What's now Barbara's room was once an illicit weapons factory. This is the sort of culture, perhaps, that led the NRA to base its headquarters just down the road. When Elmer saw it, the room was packed wall-to-ceiling with wood, metal, and black powder. "You hand that fella a lump of wood, and he'd make you the most beautiful stock. Like a master carpenter. Just as skilled a blacksmith, too. Had the only three-sided muzzle I ever did see. And a hundred twenty-three was just the long guns. Not counting the pistols or knives."

"Guy had some firepower."

"He surely did."

"Like he was indeed stocking up for the Apocalypse."

"Maybe he was. But who knows? It's a sight easier mining coal from a mile deep with your hands than divining the intentions of your average West Virginian.

"One day, not long after I bought the place and the fella'd moved back to West Virginia, I come home and there's a note, pinned to my front door."

Like all good storytellers, Elmer likes audience participation. "What'd it say, Elmer?"

"Bobo," it says, "need me a shotgun. Fast. Jimbo."

"Bobo. Jimbo. No kidding?"

"No, sir. Bobo had him a still, too. Out back. He carted the contraption away with him, but I could tell what was there, from the marks on the ground: hardware—brackets and such—on the tree trunks, foliage kilt by spilt white lightning."

## NOVEMBER 26

Ellen's demise disrupts the Hensleys' Thanksgiving Day plans, so luckily I manage to snag the last cooked turkey (with all the trimmings), desserts, etc., at the same Wegmans where Bob enjoyed his last crab soup. When I arrive at the house, Ellen is fast asleep. So is Elmer. But Barbara is up, and we have a great long chat.

She is really brilliant. Somehow we get onto the topic of St. Paul, and I tell her I'm loving this book I'm reading by a Quaker scholar who began with a very negative view of Paul but, once she went back to the original Aramaic and Greek, discovered that his words had been badly misconstrued.

"Not just badly," she says, "deliberately. They've got to tear down Paul, see, for his credentials are so impressive: student of Gamaliel, Roman citizen, murderer of Steven."

Her intelligence isn't confined to Scripture, however. Like Elmer, her big brain ranges far and wide. She loves history, for instance, as well as sociology. I'd wager she knows more about the eight U.S. presidents born in Virginia than most members of the history faculties at William and Mary, UVA, and Virginia Tech.

But her favorite figure is no Founding Father or Church Father but her own mother, related to which Barbara recounts my favorite Hensley story of all. Just before graduating the fifth grade, one of Ellen's students was diagnosed with terminal leukemia. "The poor thing.

Now, Momma loved her summer vacations, as it allowed her to do so many things she couldn't do during the school year. Bake pies, make preserves, can vegetables."

All of a sudden Elmer's with us—my guess, awakened by the thought of pies being baked. "Best apple pie in Virginia!"

Barbara nods, with conviction. "But just before her summer break begins, Momma happens upon the boy. As she's heading out for the summer, she hears him crying, tucked away, alone in a dark classroom.

"'There, there, child,' Momma says. 'What's the matter? Why aren't you *happy*? School's out. You're free! It's summertime.'

"That's when he tells her. And it just about broke Momma's big heart. See, the little boy's crying not because he's got cancer. He's done crying about that. Cried his eyes out. He's crying because he hadn't graduated the fifth grade; elementary school. Being so sick, he missed too many days of school. What this precious thing wants is to stand before our Lord as a middle schooler!"

"Amen!" say Elmer. "How blessed are the children! Now that's faith!"

Barbara smiles. "So 'course Momma's heart plum melts. She abandons her summer plans and teaches the boy, one-on-one."

Elmer briefly pouts, before breaking into a big, indulgent smile. "Not so many pies that summer!"

"Just before he dies," Barbara concludes, "the boy completes his elementary school coursework. He enters Heaven as a middle schooler. That's Momma in a nutshell."

"That's my bride!"

## NOVEMBER 28

By this point, Ellen's teaching days seem numbered. As is often the case with Alzheimer's, once it passes a tipping point the descent is rapid. Ellen isn't eating, because she can't remember what purpose food serves or how to swallow. If and when she does ingest anything, her bowels and bladder act of their own accord. Infections spring up in her mouth and elsewhere, one of which leads to pneumonia. I report,

Patient asleep. No movement whatsoever. Third time since returning from hospital . . . Fifth straight time asleep, unresponsive, including hospital.

## DECEMBER 2

I'm out of town. Barbara calls me. She's beside herself. "Momma's passed."

But through the crying and sniffling I sense happiness, too, and relief—that the ordeal is finally over. "Momma's in a better place. And she went out in a blaze of glory!"

Ellen's final seventy-two hours were especially manic. Her up-in-the-middle-of-the-night antics exhaust everyone. Elmer and Barbara don't sleep a wink until Ellen's shipped back to the hospital, where she quietly passes.

## DECEMBER 4

The memorial service is wonderful. Tributes pour in from near and far.

My favorite is from a West Virginian who grew up with Ellen. The lanky man is wearing well-worn and faded but respectfully pressed and clean overalls, with a red kerchief tucked in the back pocket. The untamable cowlick sprouting up from the right side of his head is balanced by the black patch over his left eye. He tells how he's driven long and hard to make the service. "I'd a driven to the ends of the earth. Ellen was solid as the Rock of Ages. She never judged no one. I never heard her say a single bad word 'bout nobody."

Then it's the pastor's turn. He talks about how Ellen anchored the church choir. About what a great pianist she was. Always willing to help others. Never too busy to tutor someone after school. To stay late for choir practice to help someone learn some sheet music. To come in early before Sunday School, to reconcile Luke and James the Just.

I've called Elmer several times but can't get him or Barbara. I'm worried. He fought so hard on Ellen's behalf, loved her so keenly and

completely . . . I'm worried her passing might break him. So one afternoon I drive forty-five minutes, hoping to catch them . . . but the only
one home is the annoying owl, under whose plaster feet I tuck a note:

> Elmer, I hope you're doing OK. Please give me a call.

> —Eric

## DECEMBER 19

But he doesn't call, so I head over again, unannounced. This time Elmer's home . . . in the driveway . . . apparently in a predicament.

As I pull up, his son, grandson, and a friend are milling about. They
look very frustrated, and very unhappy.

But not Elmer. He looks like his turnip's just won the blue ribbon at
the county fair. Seated in one of his many jalopies, his fingers grip the
wheel like he's ready to roll. But he'll not be rolling any time soon. The
carport's collapsed on top of him, brought down by one of the wicked
windstorms that frequent this part of Virginia.

I park, shake my head, and call out, "Elmer! You're in a bit of a
pickle!"

"Ha! I love pickles!"

## MARCH 25, 2011

I've only seen Elmer sporadically over the past sixteen months. Though
he lives forty-five minutes from me, it's but a ten-minute detour from
two new patients. However, as my new patients are less mobile and
more alone, without Elmer's support system of family and friends, I
don't feel so bad . . . preferring to allocate my limited time to where it
appears most needed. But I think about Elmer every day.

Most of the time when I am able to pop by for a visit I find him trying to mask his leg and lower-back pain. He's one tough grunt: his pill
bottles appear untouched, and he seems as active as ever: tending to his

garden, chopping his wood, pulling his red wagon. But every so often the pain blows through his defensive perimeter: he clutches his back, winces, moans.

It took me a while, but I finally got him to agree to let me take him to see my internist, but only after some horse-trading. He'd see my internist, provided I rewarded him afterward with a late lunch of biscuits and gravy; his favorite meal, forbidden by his internist. So off we head along I-66, into D.C., to see my friend David Patterson, MD.

Elmer's pain is chronic in part because Big Insurance has been stonewalling him regarding coverage. I knew Patterson could pry a Yes from the nattering nabobs of healthcare negativism, what with his doctoring half of Capitol Hill, if not also (for all I knew) the secretary of health and human services. I also knew the two brilliant bumpkins would hit it off, big time. One mightn't think so, based on what met the eye: the fastest white butcher in the country, for whom Lee's surrender at Appomattox Courthouse was one of history's darkest days; the most sought-after internist in the world's most important city (tied with his partner, Bryan Arling), who just happened to be black. I knew they'd bond because both had suffered—and overcome with a jaunty joviality—their own brand of Appalachian adversity, such as David's having to scrap with a gazillion feisty siblings to earn his keep and victuals in bum-F-bomb Kentucky, under the discriminating eye of a momma from the John Brown School of Parenting, and having to endure a downpour of bigotry on his first day of first grade as the only black kid, exacerbated by his being, far and away, the smartest urchin in his hardscrabble patch of bluegrass. "I'll never forget it," I'll never forget David telling me, "I was drenched." I'd responded, "Bad rainstorm, huh?" He'd shaken his head. "Spit-storm, from all my classmates spitting on me."

Following introductions, David and Elmer disappear into an exam room, while I return to the reception area. Thirty minutes later, even from a ways away, I can hear them hooting and hollering like time's stood still. But my schedule's not so relaxed, so I get up, walk over, pound on the door, and holler my own self: "FOR PETE'S SAKE! What're y'all *doin'* in there!? Got a still in there?!" Soon they emerge, their faces like those of kids having been caught raiding the cookie jar, not the least bit ashamed, wishing they'd had more time to gorge on their mutual good humor, and wreck my schedule. Though David writes a great letter on his behalf, I never hear back from Elmer.

## JUNE 23

Elmer's church also gives him the runaround. One day, he asks if I might help him with a legal issue. By the sound of it, some petty bureaucrats in his denomination's version of Vatican City are confounding him with legalese regarding a trust he'd established, that involved the church selling some land and Barbara (and/or Lake) having the right to occupy his rambler while alive. "Sure," I say, "I'm happy to try and help. You got some papers I can take a look at?"

"I'll have Lake send them to you."

My assumption is that the amount is maybe in the $25,000 range, $125,000 tops, given what I'd guess the rambler to be worth and the used car lot that surrounds it. After all, he'd been a meat-cutter, not a hedge-fund manager. The rambler's very modest, its furnishings spare.

"By the way, what're we talking about here, Elmer? How much money'd you give to your church? "

"A few million dollars."

"And they're jerking you around?"

He laughs, not snidely. "Funny, isn't it?"

## JULY 15

While in Florence, Italy, with my wife, my phone rings. My first thought is one of worry, related to my kids or parents.

"Is this Eric?"

"Yes."

"This is Pam Hensley, Lake's wife?"

"Hello, Pam. How are you?"

"I'm okay, thanks. But . . . I'm not sure you've heard?"

It doesn't appear so. "What's going on? Gosh I hope everything's okay with Elmer . . . ?"

"Yes, yes—well, he's just really, really sad. Barbara's just passed."

"Oh . . . I am so sorry!"

## FEBRUARY 6, 2012

The Grim Reaper prefers to strike while I'm overseas. More than half of my patients die while I'm abroad, even though I only travel internationally maybe six weeks a year.

This time it's Elmer. I'd visited him in the hospital just prior to leaving for Europe. He was in great spirits. He had everyone in stitches, especially the nurses, the day before he died.

Lake reaches me in Warsaw. "Daddy passed two days ago. His heart just gave out."

"It was a mighty big heart," I say.

"Yes, it was."

Elmer also had a mighty big funny bone. I'll never forget his laughing at the fidgety squirrels and cackling crows that greeted him the day I'd shuttled him over to my place, because he wanted to pay his respects to some of the largest white oaks and black walnuts in Virginia, arrayed throughout my antebellum farm. The tree he loved most, however, was our tall tulip-poplar, given its peculiar double-trunk formation. I can still see him chuckling, his hand resting at the base of the wishbone, staring up into the fall leaves, bursting in yellow, orange, and red.

Like my dad is, still, I am, and most country folk are, Elmer was an early riser. He never lectured me, but, like his teacher-bride, he taught me nonetheless that while the writings of Thomas Berry, Thoreau, and St. Francis *about* Brother Squirrel, Sister Deer, and the Holy Outdoors are wonderful, what such spiritual counselors would most counsel is not reading, but—venturing outdoors. So I'm doing much more venturing out these days . . . hiking and kayaking with my wife . . . opening my soul to Gaia's sights, sounds, smells, breezy touch, and overall rhythm . . . whether along Kauai's Na Pali Coast or in Virginia's Piedmont.

I've been very fortunate to have traveled to many of the world's loveliest cities and towns . . . staying in some amazing accommodations . . . marveling at architectural masterpieces and works of art . . . yet all this man-made stuff and orchestration pales in comparison to what happens every morning in my Blue Ridge backyard: when the lustrous constellations dim . . . as the moon gets ready to hand things over to the sun . . . when that first birdsong enlivens the silence . . .

These days, I typically meditate each morning, outside, just before dawn . . . and, thanks to Elmer, I've come to appreciate how each day I'm blessed with my own personally composed and performed Daily Special Symphony . . . maybe with the gobbling Tom turkey as Yo-Yo Ma, or the warbling mockingbird as Anne-Sophie Mutter . . . but always with the same Maestro.

Elmer loved his sunsets, too. Now I do. With the light pollution from the Nation's Capital not reaching me, I see why another Chicago law school grad (named Hubble) preferred (along with his friend Einstein) staring agog into the night sky, at the ever-expanding magnificence of billions of galaxies and trillions of stars—to racking up thousands of billable hours . . . The owls hooting an amicus brief in accompaniment to the brightening rheostat of our Milky Way . . . that makes the lighted kitsch of Times Square or Hong Kong seem downright pathetic . . . and guides our resident momma turkey, as she shepherds her hatchlings from the dense woods.


My own momma grew up in the great outdoors. Swimming in Sherwood Forest in Maryland. Attending college in Lynchburg, Virginia, in the heart of the Blue Ridge Mountains.

But she hates being outdoors in Florida. "It's so flat and featureless. So hot. There's never any breeze. I can't wait to get back home."

"Home?" I say, as I detect an edge to her tone. "You mean come April?"

"No. I mean for good. Your father and I appreciate all the work you, your brothers, and sister did in moving us to the new place, but it's just not what we want. We don't like it here. We're moving back to Maryland, to Fox Hill. For good. It's time."

My siblings and I'd assumed we'd had it all figured out. In moving our parents to an assisted-living community, we thought they'd be safe, secure, surrounded by a peer group with whom they could relate, and they could still golf in Florida when it got cold in D.C.

But in trying to be a caregiver to my parents, I've violated two of Rosalie's tips: *Don't expect your patients to conform to your standards or expectations*, and *Don't assume you know what their needs or feelings are*. My bad.

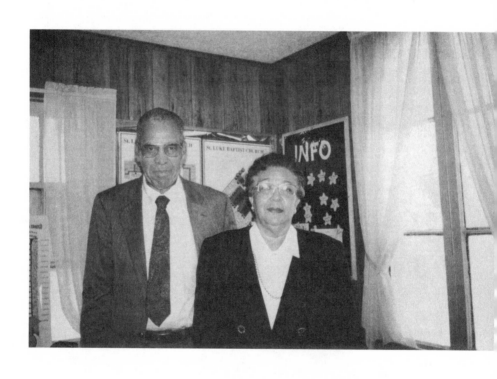

# OWNERSHIP ISN'T ALL THAT IT'S CRACKED UP TO BE

I continue flirting with assumptions. Despite some glitches with my octogenarian parents, based on my experiences with Bob (who's passed) and the Hensleys (at this time all three are still very much alive), I assume I've got the hang of hospice. Then reality sets in.

Cecilia Tull is ninety-four. I visit her assisted-living apartment thirty-three times—that is, more than twice as often as I do Bob Zimmerman and Ellen Hensley combined. Cecilia rarely talks to me, never smiles at me, hardly ever looks at me. The few times our eyes do connect—she jerks hers away as if mine are radioactive and repellant. (I often leave with Simon & Garfunkel's "Cecilia" playing in my head.)

Being a glutton for punishment, I add another patient onto my roster: Moses Besht. It's clear when I first lay eyes on him that I'll never dream of calling him anything but "Mr. Besht," or "Sir." His face is a war zone of two raw, zealous emotions, manifest most strikingly in his veiny brown eyes: anger and sadness. The former he seems to have husbanded and marinated in bile especially for my benefit, as if I were yet another czarist thug, about to unleash another pogrom against his harmless shtetl, situated along the river border that once separated Poland and Ukraine (when both were still ruled by the Romanovs). Almost a century old, Moses looks like he's lived every minute of it—hard. Things he's not worked so hard, apparently, in addition to his smile, are his vocal cords. He's even less talkative than Cecilia. I visit him religiously for three months, and not once does he utter so much as one word to me. Though not Jewish, several of my best friends are. I tell him this, as well as how much I love reading Hillel and Heschel, Buber and Wiesel. My attempt at connectedness provokes him all the more. I ask the head RN at his nursing home if he can talk. She nods. "He just chooses not to. He's a cranky old cuss, isn't he?" So, week after week, visit upon visit, this Aaron-less Moses just sits and smolders, staring out the window or off into the corner of the room. He does, however, scribble notes every now and again, grunting as he pokes me with his mini-missives, like he's The Donald and I'm the lamest-ever hospice apprentice; querying if I've seen his family, or know when (not if) they'll be arriving. As I've never spoken with let alone met any of his tribe, but do know they seldom visit (the worse angels of my nature whispering, "Big surprise"), I do my best to deflect and dance around the topic. When one day Moses gesticulates towards the closet, growling and scribbling that some thief stole his cardigan, clearly suggesting that a good old-school stoning was called for, I buy him a new one. He not so much ignores my gift as takes it as evidence that I'm the thief. Meanwhile, he totally ignores the flowers and food I sometimes bring him.

By way of thanks I contract sepsis, which homes in on my bum eye. My docs can't be sure, but they think I either picked it up at Cecilia's assisted-living facility or Moses's nursing home. No good deed goes unpunished. Now I'm the one bedridden . . . for months . . . nursing my left eye, which, after having undergone sixteen operations since 1993, is forming and popping countless blisters every day, atop and around the transplanted cornea that my body's rejected.

As my doctor forbids me from setting foot in another nursing home or assisted-living facility, I don't even get the chance personally to say good-bye to Moses or Cecilia. (I send cards and candy.) Had I done so, maybe then Moses would have piped up: "I never wanted you here anyway! Your replacement sweater is shoddy, by the way. Your flowers, dead. Your food, stale. Good riddance!"

I actually would have welcomed such an outburst. It would have brought a smile to my face. His too, I like to think.

My caregiving smiles remain in drought for some time. But at least another round of surgery at Washington Hospital Center remedies my eyes-blisters (for the most part), so I'm ready to step up to the volunteer plate again.

Rosalie assigns me a patient who's suffering from an especially nasty form of cancer—pancreatic—that, once it presents, often results in a super-quick death. In the prime of her life, just named partner at a top D.C. law firm, the woman suddenly finds herself staring death in the face. She'll leave behind her parents, husband, and several children. I'm told she might last two months, tops.

All those late nights and formidable billable hours, foregone fun and family time—for what? I really want to help. Rosalie thinks I can, being a lawyer, about the same age. But the newly minted partner-patient wants none of me; perhaps, I muse, because my being a member of The Bar, too, would highlight something she'd just as soon forget. She ignores my phone calls, rejects me, and—poor Esquire—doesn't last long.

After batting away my suggestion that I'm in any way at fault for my string of hospice debacles, Rosalie assigns me another patient. "This young Indian woman came to the D.C. area just a year ago, her megabright husband drawn to the high-tech sector, aspiring to be the next Indian billionaire, Bangalore's version of Bill Gates." But, unbeknownst to her, she arrived carrying the HIV virus. "Now it's full-blown AIDS. Most likely, she got it from her husband, but he exhibits no symptoms. It's such a sad situation!" Rosalie says the woman's impoverished family was against her emigrating. Now her husband's wealthy family has shunned her, too, shamed by her condition, and regarding her as a threat—as well as an insult—to their Golden Boy, who's rarely at home, consumed 24/7 by his IPO road show. While he's wining and dining with Masters of the Universe, she's all alone at home, bags protruding from her body, processing waste. Her once-lovely, full figure is now emaciated, pocked with lesions that seep purulent discharge.

But the IPO's a huge success.

"Rosalie! That's so tragic! Can I think about it a day or two?"

"Sure," she says. "Take your time. This is a tough one, I know."

I confer with other caregivers, volunteers as well as pros. They all wave red flags. The incredibly compassionate Maureen Samet says, "If I didn't have to? I wouldn't visit her. That sounds awful. Maybe I'm a bad person. But she's got open sores, for goodness sake. She'll not be with us for long, poor dear. But I'm married, got kids, and want to be around for a while. So, though I'm sure it hurts her feelings, and it pricks my conscience, I wear gloves. I've got to think of my own family and my other patients. I just don't feel safe."

So I'm facing a moral dilemma. I'm not sure whether to take on this patient. I too am married, with a wife, kids, parents. If an experienced and compassionate RN is hesitant and fearful, shouldn't I be, also?

Perhaps. But I call the AIDS sufferer nonetheless, several times. There's never any answer. (Which doesn't mean she's not home . . . listening to me, trying to decide whether to pick up . . . whether she should be ashamed . . . whether her parents, in-laws, and apparently even her AWOL husband are all right . . . that, somehow, she's to blame). I leave messages saying things like "I'd like to meet you" and "Please give me a call." But I'm a liar. I'd really rather not meet her. I really hope she doesn't call me.

Rosalie does. "She's passed."


## NOVEMBER 13, 2009

Rosalie calls again. She's nothing if not persistent. (No wonder she's tripled the number of volunteers in less than two years.) "I know you're still helping out the Hensley family, and you've experienced some bumps in the road as of late, but I'm just wondering . . . I've just been contacted by another family that lives near you."

"Just wondering? . . ."

"First, how's your eye?"

"Much better, thanks. My last operation really helped. I'm good to go."

"You sure?"

"I'm sure."

"Remember my tips during orientation and training!"

"Which one?"

"*Don't* number one!"

"*Don't visit if you're sick.*"

"And number six?"

"*Don't take on too many patients.* Got it. I'm good. Really. What've you got for me?"

"I've only had one brief chat, so my workup is a little thin. Patient's name is Gordon Ford. He's seventy-three—"

"Same as Bob Zimmerman."

"Good memory. I'd forgotten. Anyway, Gordon's lived his entire life in and around Marshall, Upperville, et cetera."

"Horse country."

"Exactly. And, in fact, that's been his line of work—horses. That and gardening."

"Interesting mix."

"Interesting employer, too: Paul Mellon."

"I'll say."

"Patient lives with his wife in Marshall. I've only spoken with his daughter, Yolanda Mason, who lives in Berryville. Yolanda was having trouble keeping it together over the phone.

"Her father suffers from advanced congestive heart disease, bordering on total failure. His kidneys are failing. He's very weak, eating no solid food, on oxygen. It's a full code situation—DNR. He's been prescribed morphine, but he's refused to take it under any circumstances."

"Poor guy . . ."

"Yes. Very sad."

"Things have a way of piling on, don't they?"

"Yes they do. But the family has a strong faith. Though Yolanda describes her father as being 'more spiritual than religious,' she also—I made a note of this—said he's the lead usher at one of the two churches he and his wife attend regularly."

In addition to Yolanda, Mr. Ford has one other child, also a daughter, as well as five grandchildren and three great-grandchildren. He and his wife, Dorothy, have been married for fifty years. "Yolanda hopes you might be able to provide companionship not only for her father but also for her mother, who, she says, is also very lonely."

"Help her . . . how? Any specifics?"

"Run errands . . . to the grocery store, that sort of thing. Mrs. Ford doesn't drive."

"Okay. Sounds pretty simple."

There I go assuming again!

## NOVEMBER 14

Pellam Court is a far cry from Rokeby, Paul Mellon's four-thousand-acre spread just up the road, whose thoroughbred stables have produced more than one thousand stakes winners. Each unit in the Fords' townhome complex has an assigned parking space, stenciled on the curb, but as it's a Saturday and people are off work, there are no vacancies, anywhere, so I'm forced to park out in the street. The front steps are blanketed not in Kentucky bluegrass but Monsanto Astroturf. Stiff bristles poke through the worn soles of my Topsiders. There's no bell. I rap on the screen door.

"*Landy*??" a woman hollers. "Someone at the door!"

The door is answered by Yolanda, the elder of Gordon Ford's two daughters. A mocha-skinned African American in her late thirties or early forties, she says nothing as she nods, shakes my hand, and steps to the side so I can enter.

Once the door closes behind me, two related impressions jump out: cleanliness and orderliness. The former on account of Dorothy's having cleaned house for forty-four years, the latter on account of Gordon's having tended, for fifty-two years, the greenhouse for one of the world's wealthiest men, whose designs were borrowed both by Jackie O, in creating the Rose Garden, and by Versailles, in renovating the great French gardens, which, until Paul Mellon and Gordon Ford weighed in, had gone to seed. There are no seeds in evidence here. Surfaces shine, windows are streakless, knickknacks are all in their proper place, atop lace doilies. Humble wall hangings are perfectly spaced and aligned.

"Why, hello," says Dorothy, as she hobbles from her kitchen. In her early seventies (I guess), her hue is a shade lighter than Yolanda. Her eyes twinkle behind her glasses as we shake hands. "Please," she says, "have a seat. Set a spell." She's not about to forward some stranger to her dying husband without at least a little bit of face-to-face vetting.

I sit in the corner in an easy chair: the hot seat. Dorothy sits to my right with the perfect posture that's always eluded Cotillion-trained me. Yolanda's on the couch, opposite me, across the gleaming coffee table.

The thawing November Saturday has speckled my shoes and jeans with mud, which must be like fingernails on a chalkboard to my fastidious hostess. But Dorothy says nothing. The three us just sit for a moment, eyeing each other, smiling, catching a breath. From what Rosalie's told me, tranquility has been rare of late, so probably Dorothy wants to make the most of it. After a minute or so she starts in. "Thank you for coming by."

"My pleasure."

"My husband's just got back from the hospital. Can't do no more for him down there."

"I'm very sorry."

She shuts her eyes for a moment, then nods. "Thank you. He's been in and out of the hospital for, oh, the better part of a year."

"Three years, Momma," says Yolanda.

By the quick, sharp look Dorothy casts Yolanda's way, interrupting one's elders was rarely brooked in the Ford household. But Dorothy lets this interruption slide. "Three. But them times they thought they could do something. Not this time."

"Daddy's got COPD. Been having problems breathing for years. But now it's really bad. He—" Gordon's favorite daughter chokes up, out of breath herself.

Yolanda's abrupt exhalation triggers a yawn in Dorothy. Based on Rosalie's briefing, coupled with my hospice experiences hitherto, mother and daughter both appear to be flat-out exhausted . . .

From want of sleep and the relentless emotional siege, as the stoic husband and father attempts, but fails, to fully stifle his moaning, wailing, and whimpering or confine his blank stares to times when no one's looking.

From the 911 calls and the fretting: will the Rescue Squad arrive in time?? From the frenzied sorties to Fauquier Hospital, fifteen miles south. From the guilt of—sometimes, when especially depleted—secretly harboring the hope that Mercy will intervene and Company 8 won't arrive in time. Allowing Gordon to rest in peace.

From the phone ringing off the hook. The neighbors constantly traipsing through, provisioning enough homemade stew and cornbread to feed an army. The pastor's well-meaning bromides. Everyone fumbling, struggling with what to say and do.

Me, especially. "I'm so very sorry."

"Thank you," they both say, simultaneously.

"Please tell me how I might be able to help."

They don't respond. Other than to look at each other.

Rosalie told me Dorothy simply wants a few hours every now and again so she might escape to the store, the dentist, the hairdresser, her own doctors.

Finally the expectant widow says something. "I'm hoping you can help me, us, figure out something Gordon wants. He won't ask for nothing. Not for his'self, anyway. All he's concerned about is that I'm provided for—after he's gone. That's Gordon for you. Thinking about everyone but his'self. Except yesterday, right, Landy?"

"Right, Momma."

"Being so short of breath, it's hard for Gordon to talk, but last night he asked Landy to try and find him a Dreamsicle."

"That takes me back," I say. How poignant the choice in food. I'm reminded of Ellen Hensley's love of ice cream, Bob Zimmerman's of pancakes and crab soup. Last Suppers, breakfasts, and other food seem a common element on many Bucket Lists.

"Gordon loves his Dreamsicles! But Landy couldn't find none. Nowheres. Finally, she do. When she's back home, I ask Gordon if he'd like his Dreamsicle. He says, 'Bring it on.'"

"Bring it on," I parrot, looking over at Yolanda. "Wonderful. Well done."

Yolanda smiles, shyly.

"Now, young man . . . you bring it on. Where're your people from? How old are you?"

"Fifty-one."

"Why, you young!" The word *young* sails away and trails off, like a kite suddenly seized by a gust of wind. She follows with questions about my wife, kids, where we live, etc.

"Done a lot of living in my fifty-one years."

Her lips purse as her eyes move to the narrow corridor leading from the kitchen, by the bathroom . . . a knot having formed around a preacher, maneuvering his corpulence in an attempt to let people pass without spilling the victuals sagging his paper plate. I count more than a dozen people milling about: up and down the stairs, visiting her husband; dropping off food or eating it; waiting in line to freshen up. The entirely African American crowd (save for me) includes the couple's granddaughter from New York, fellow Methodist congregants, and neighbors.

With such an apparently vibrant support system, I wonder: Why do they need me? What do I bring to the table? Were I a doctor, nurse, or preacher, okay, but I'm just someone offering generic "companion care," and the Fords sure don't seem to lack caring companions.

When Dorothy's eyes return to me, she says, "Gordon's in bad shape. Awful pain. But he don't never complain."

Once she pauses, I weigh in. "What days are best for you? What're some of the things your husband likes? What do you think he wants from me? Wants me to do while I'm here?"

"I hope he tells you! Because he won't tell me. Every time I ask him what he wants, he turns it back around on me, to say, 'All I want is for you to be taken care of, darling. Because you're my prize carnation.'"

"Carnation?"

"Gordon's favorite flower is a white carnation. Mr. Paul Mellon has his'self flowers that cost—oh good Lord, more than you can believe. But Gordon prefers just a white carnation."

"What a wonderful story. And a wonderful testament to you. I know, from now on, I'll never think of a white carnation the same."

She mulls over my compliment, momentarily (I suppose plumbing for sincerity), then smiles and wags her head toward the stairs. "Well, I guess you can go on up and meet him now." She hollers, for all to hear, "Hospice man's coming on up now. Make way!"

Compliance is immediate. People pour down the stairs, squeeze into the kitchen, stream out the front door. A lovely black lady—whose elegant magenta hat is accented by a white feather, angled stylishly—sneaks a peek at me, and I'm suddenly self-conscious, not at being the sole Caucasian but at being so shabbily and muddily attired.

"He's expecting you," Dorothy says to me.

I thought she'd be joining me. I want her to. But her eyes say, *Never had much time or use for training wheels around here.* She doesn't move a muscle.

So off I go, navigating around the curious neighbors and my curdling anxiety about what lay in store. I clear a traffic jam on the stairs and duck, so as not to crack my skull on the low-slung ceiling, and finally arrive at Gordon's second-floor room.

I rap on the open door and step inside. The bedroom's as neat and clean as the rest of the home. As neat and clean as possible, that is, what with tidy sacks holding bodily waste.

Gordon seems larger than life. He just about fills up the entire room: he's so tall, the room so small. His feet resemble snorkel flippers—heels dangling over the edge of the bed. He's hooked up to all sorts of tubes and devices, befitting his congestive heart failure, kidney failure, and other virulently opportunistic ailments.

Yet he seems at ease. His eyes twinkle like his wife's. (Though he wears no glasses.) Such luminosity the refracted essence, perhaps, of the kindred spirit that's sustained them through the ordinary pitch and yaw of a long married life, let alone their current trials and tribulations.

And his smile is much more expressive than Dorothy's. Rubbery almost. Peculiarly so.

"Hello, Mr. Ford," I begin. "Pleasure to meet you." For some reason, I feel I ought not simply presume to shake this man's hand, any more than I should poke the Blue Period Picasso his employer gifted to the National Gallery of Art. So I keep my distance, taking a seat in a rigid cane-backed chair, kitty-corner from his bed. We're a few feet from one another.

"Pleasure to meet you," he responds. Then he giggles. It's weird, both the sound and the sight. This large man, on the brink of death— giggling. I've seen some odd things during my hospice work, but this takes the cake. Then, as his eyes pass over me, I think I understand the levity: he's imagining the reaction downstairs of his black family and formally dressed friends to the strange white man in the filthy blue jeans.

Mr. Ford is my eleventh patient, and, as always, I'm unsure how to proceed, what to say or do. It's always improv. My first few minutes bomb, or so it seems. I know it's hard for him to speak, but his look seems half stare, half glare. The levity's sure long gone. His head lay angled on his pillow, adding to the impression that he's studying me, like an anthropologist.

I muddle along, fidget, shift in my seat, comment on the weather, this and that.

His only reaction is to open and close his lips, almost fish-like.

I ask, "Some TV maybe?"

His pinched smile acts as a levee, fending off a frown. *Son, I infer, you're not too bright, are you? I'm about to kick the bucket, and you think I want to look at some trash on TV?*

As suggested by Rosalie during training, refined by her briefing, I've brought some reading material, including a Bible, which I hold up. "Like me to read something?"

He shakes his head, no—politely, but unequivocally.

Okay, now what? As I take a deep breath, I notice a photo across the room, beside the TV. I rise, step over, and have a look. "Who's this? Handsome."

Gordon's face brightens. He takes a pull of oxygen, then, with some effort, speaks. "Grandson. Demetrius. Running back. High School."

Yeah! "Fauquier High?"

"Clarke County." His pride is palpable. As much as any father, or grandfather, of any Super Bowl MVP.

The ice now broken, after some further sputtering on my part, our conversation ambles along. But it's still mostly me asking questions, interspersed with his smiling or replying with yes, no, or short answers. This big man isn't big on words, but I do learn that he met Dorothy at a dance hall in Middleburg . . . that he's worked for Paul Mellon the same number of years that he's been married (fifty-three) . . . and that Dorothy got him the job through a friend.

"I understand you've spent time around horses."

He nods, slightly. Humbly. (Rather than boast about being around scores of the world's finest thoroughbreds.)

I ramble, nervously. "My wife was big into horses. Rode with Warrenton Hunt. She quit because she got thrown a few times, had some bad fractures, and, the nail in the coffin? A friend of ours—a great rider—died on account of her mount stepping into a groundhog hole."

Nail in the coffin?? Did I really just say that?? What an idiot!

Why am I the anxious one here? I'm not the one on (or near) my deathbed. I try salvaging the situation by rambling some more. "My wife grew up in Ireland. Imprisoned in a high-walled convent school run by tyrannical nuns. Ellen prayed every day—for her own horse. So she could jump the wall and gallop away."

A smile stretches his gaunt cheeks.

Yeah . . . "I've just popped by today to make your acquaintance, and it's been a real pleasure. I'll stay much longer next time. Your wife, daughter, and I figure this coming Tuesday's a good time for me to return. That sound okay?"

He doesn't answer.

"When I return, what would you like to do?"

Not much, it seems.

I've lost the connection. His mind's retreated. Somewhere far away. But I hack about, extemporizing, throwing out possibilities. Something I might bring. Something we might do together. Probing for some bridge of rapport.

But with slow shakes of his head, he professes to be entirely content. Even though from Rosalie I know he's in terrible physical pain, let alone the psychic fear of the unknown.

I rise from my chair, defeated. "Well . . . I'll see you in a few days, I guess. Okay?"

His eyes flicker. A slight shrug jostles the bedsheets.

Despite his withdrawal, for some reason I now get the feeling that touching him would no longer be presumptuous or invasive, so I place my hand on his broad, bony shoulder, then slip down and clasp his limp hand. We don't shake. Don't even squeeze. Just cling.

"See you Tuesday, Mr. Ford. A real pleasure meeting you." Looking into his eyes, now I squeeze his hand.

He reciprocates—meets my eyes, returns the squeeze. "Pleasure meeting you."

Yeah! When I'm by the door, my back to him, one foot in the hallway, he asks—his voice soft, reedy, slightly high-pitched—"Got any horse books?"

I pause. Turn around. "Horse books?"

He looks embarrassed. Like his modest request might be putting me out.

"I'll see. If so, I'll bring it, or them, next time. I'm really looking forward to our next visit together, Mr. Ford."

His smile is subdued.


Later that same Saturday, a little before 4 P.M., I head up to my barn in search of this horse book my wife was given when she rode with the

Warrenton Hunt and our barn was home to several high-spirited thoroughbreds. Since my wife gave up riding and donated her mounts to charity, and it's clear the humans have decamped, our barn's gotten a bit out of hand. But, mercifully, the only evidence of the Wild Kingdom is what's left of a possum, in the middle of the aisle.

In the tack room, atop an antebellum farm table, I find *The Magnificent Horse*. Its glossy pages are filled with photos. There's a rearing steed on the cover. Great!

## NOVEMBER 16

But too late.

I notice I've got a voicemail. It's Rosalie. "Mr. Ford passed away at one thirty this morning. I knew you'd want to know."

## NOVEMBER 17

I return as planned to the Ford home, even though my patient has died.

Dorothy greets me at the door. She's much less subdued than when we first met. "I'm so sorry!" She reaches over and touches my shoulder.

She's sorry? . . .

"I wanted to tell you not to bother coming. But I lost your number." Her voice still twills, but today there's more relief, a tone of—liberation.

Like you haven't had enough on your plate! Her being so considerate knots my throat. I hand her the heavy book. "Your husband asked if I had any horse books. My wife had one, but she and I both wanted your husband to have it. We thought you might want it, still."

"I didn't know! Aren't you thoughtful! Gordon sure loved his horses. Here . . . " She walks over to her favorite chair, beckoning me. "Have a seat."

"You sure? You must—"

"Have a seat."

I do as I'm told.

"Gordon passed quietly. At peace. We was holding hands. Not long before he died, I see him staring in the corner of the room, intently.

'What is it, Gordon?' I say. He points. 'Angels,' he says. 'You don't see 'em?' I look. I don't see anything. When I look back at him, he smiles and says—the very last thing he says—'I'm ready to step on board that train.' Then he was gone."

Any response from me seeming so utterly lame, I demur.

"Couldn't ask for no better husband. Knowing he'll be waiting for me keeps me strong."

"Mrs. Ford—"

"Please, call me Dorothy."

"Alright. Dorothy, your husband seemed like such a brave, lovely man. His smile and mirthful chuckle, especially, I'll never forget."

"Oh, he had a sense of humor, alright. He sure liked to laugh."

"I've really enjoyed getting to know you, too. And Yolanda. I'd like very much to visit you from time to time, if that's okay?"

"Oh, that'd be lovely."

Over the next month, I ring her several times. Either she's out, asleep, or electing not to pick up the phone.


## DECEMBER 15

I wouldn't do this in every situation—not even most. But based on my visit with Dorothy four weeks prior, and my sense that she's not the type who likes to put people out, I decide to pop by for an unannounced visit. I've got with me some Christmas cookies and one of Heidelberg Bakery's elaborate gingerbread houses. That the same deep maroon Buick is here as during my two prior visits doesn't say much, as Dorothy doesn't drive. I rap on the door.

"Who is it?" I hear, from somewhere inside.

I identify myself, half yelling.

"Hospice man?"

I smile. "Yes. Hospice man."

"Just a minute."

We spend half an hour together. It's wonderful. She's a lovely lady. Seeing the horse book atop the dining room table skips my heart a beat.

Thereafter, unless out of town, I typically visit her every other Sunday for an hour. She never lets me take her out to lunch, though I offer on numerous occasions. However, every now and again, on a weekday, I take her to a doctor's appointment up in Winchester, not far from River Church, where Bob's daughter copastors.

## MARCH 7, 2010

My wife and I have just returned from our first visit to Hawaii. Only able to squeeze in a four-day trip (most of my family and friends thinking me nuts, given the twenty-hour, multi-leg journey from D.C.), Ellen and I don't get off Oahu. Yet we still see and do a lot. The highlight is our visit to Shangri-La, the former home of the late Doris Duke. Right about the time Gordon began working for the world's wealthiest man, Paul Mellon, the world's wealthiest woman, Doris Duke, was putting the finishing touches on her amazing, Islamic-inspired Hawaiian home. Like so many do when they first encounter the world's most remote islands, Duke fell instantly in love. Problem was, she wasn't willing to love Hawaii on Hawaiian terms; she confused ownership with happiness. When her magnificent estate encroached on an Oahu beach that—by law—could never be owned, it wasn't the lonely billionaire but rather the thousands of humble Hawaiians who reveled in diving from her yacht slip into the Pacific. "I thought I liked to collect stuff, but that Duke lady was something else."

"What you collect?" asks Dorothy.

"Everything, just about, at one time or another." Nodding toward the horse book, I say, "I'll tell you something, finding that book was a miracle!" I go into detail about the state of our cluttered barn. "I found the book triple-decker-sandwiched between some English, French, German, and Swedish travel posters, circa the nineteen thirties, my wife and I picked up in Vancouver in the eighties, a lithograph of the Battle of Antietam that I'd traded some of my coin collection for in the seventies, and an old Indian shield acquired in Bombay—before it was officially renamed Mumbai—made out of—I've never been able to determine, definitively—elephant or rhino hide."

"Wha—aat?! Why . . . you just up to your eyeballs in stuff!"

"It's crazy, I know."

But . . . do I really know?

On the ride home, Dorothy's natural, nonjudgmental comment seeps into my thick, acquisitive skull. All my life I've been an inveterate collector of stuff. Stamps. Coins. Gold. Civil War, Cold War, and political memorabilia. Soft drink bottle caps, open-pontil bottles. Old books, maps, and posters. Religious artifacts, from Lithuanian icons to Buddhist ivories. Antique advertising. Pre-NASCAR stock-car stuff. How ridiculous, wasteful, selfish, pathetic—pathological—it all seems now . . . compared to Dorothy and me collecting our moments together . . . swapping tips on the right flower to stalk in order to glimpse the elusive, ephemeral hummingbird . . . which grocer stocks the ripest peaches . . . whether Bathsheba or Gomer was the worst harlot, Job or Ruth the most faithful God-fearer, Isaiah or Nathan the best prophet . . . and, especially, how to be a good spouse, parent, child, sibling, and friend, especially to those in need.

Once home, I head back up to the barn, take inventory, and start thinking how best to jettison all my excess stuff. I contact Kathryn Gendreau, a friend who specializes in eBay transactions, and we cut a deal that motivates her to unload as much stuff as possible, as fast as possible.

## MARCH 21

Kathryn starts racking up sales, the biggest-ticket item being a rare, framed deed signed by both Thomas Jefferson, as president, and James Madison, Jefferson's neighbor, as vice president. I'll be jettisoning for some time. How fortunate I feel . . . like Scrooge the morning after his reprieve. My wife and I delight in distributing our liquidated assets to the local food bank, her therapeutic riding program for autistic kids, our son's volunteer firehouse, and other beneficiaries . . . all far worthier than our barn's live groundhogs and dead possums.

Every now and then, however, I stumble across something that's actually worth keeping: stuff—stuffed with meaning. My most notable find is a small, molten image of Jesus. Carved from a bullet, once carried in the shirt pocket of a Civil War soldier, I know at once who'd appreciate the irony of this graven image.

But stuff is clingy. I'd always liked my Jesus bullet. It used to speak to me—of some poor kid, quaking in terror at Bull Run, having just seen a round of grapeshot turn his best bud's brains to mush.

Yet I manage to throw off the useless yoke of my materially bound recollections. Like Hawaii's lapping surf, I've logged and will forever enjoy the memory, but I don't need a scrap of metal any more than I need a conch shell to sustain the benefit. So I place a call. "Elmer?"

"Yes? Who's calling?"

"It's Eric."

He laughs, the sight and sound of which I've sorely missed. "Hello! How you been? Enjoying this weather?"

"Been trying to. Listen, you gonna be around tomorrow?"

"You obviously did all right at Iwo Jima and Okinawa without this," I say when handing over the Jesus bullet, "but . . ."

The totem looks especially tiny in Elmer's big, beefy palm. He reaches for his glasses and has a gander at his Savior. "Ain't that something?? Thank you! Hungry? Up for a turnip?"

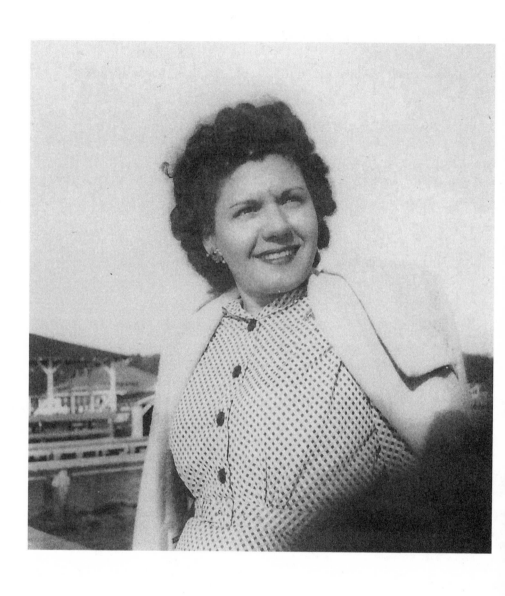

# TALK LESS, COMMUNICATE MORE

Religion plays a big role in the lives of most hospice patients, which is understandable given how faith is so rooted in questions involving the hereafter. But mixing hospice and religion can be volatile. Witness the Catholic-Protestant spat that erupted between the Zimmerman sisters just before Bob's passing.

As I was with the Zimmerman clan, caregivers are sometimes asked to mediate. But it's dicey wearing the blue helmet in such a combat zone. Several *Dos* and *Don'ts* are designed to help protect the caregiver in such instances, including not offering unsolicited advice or passing judgment. However, the focus of Rosalie's caveats are the patients, not the caregivers. Consequently, every now and then she has to fire a volunteer (if counseling fails) if and when visits veer from caregiving to converting—to Christianity, Scientology, Wicca, or whatever.

Virginia is still very religious, especially in the backcountry where I live and ply my trade as a volunteer. But the Commonwealth is no longer monolithic, even where cattle vastly outnumber people. You'll find the likes of Scots-Irish Elmer Hensley (thankfully), but such devout Christians now enjoy fellowship with African Americans like Dorothy Ford as well as not just tolerate but welcome the Muslims they see at the store, the Mormon nurses who bathe them at home, the

Bahai temple down the road, and the many "Papists," once so reviled by Virginian's early settlers. My adopted state has come a long way on the tolerance scale, which, to some extent, explains why America's first colony again voted in 2012 for a mixed-race global citizen named Barack Hussein Obama rather than the candidate ardently stumped for by both Jerry Falwell's Moral Majority and Pat Robertson's 700 Club, both of which are based in Virginia.

Rosalie said that all of the hospice *Dos* and *Don'ts* boil down to being compassionate, and, based on my experiences thus far with a dozen patients, I can see how she'd say this. But I think things can be boiled down even further, to tolerance, for tolerance is often the only soil in which compassion can take root.

My family's got its share of problems, but, fortunately, tolerance is not one of them. Religiously speaking, the Lindner family is a litter of mutts, including northern Catholics (Irish and Polish), Southern Baptists, Episcopalians, converted Mormons, murky Czech Judaic strains, and an ex-seminarian New Age guru living in an organic Scottish commune who insists that Dante's Satan is alive and well in the form of Dupont's pesticides and Monsanto's soybeans.

Based on my family's diverse proclivities, coupled with my extensive travel (forty-eight states, thirty-five countries), I've inferred that, generally speaking, Protestants prefer to brood while Catholics like to yak. But I also know that exceptions to this rule are especially entertaining.

In my family, as in many, the religious diversity distills particularly piquantly during yuletide. Our centerpiece is always the same: who's going to host the traditional, all-important Christmas brunch? As we don't get together as much as we'd like, when we do we try to make the most of it. Making the most of it turns on who'll be in town and what venue will work best. Where can my mother showcase her unique, exotic gift-locating and -matching skills and my father cook his beloved anti-cardiac kielbasa as well as serve up his whiskey sours that—like the hooch brewed in the backyard trailer by the prior resident of Elmer's place—have spent the better part of the year fermenting in Thaddeus's senior-living still? One who often wants to play host is my devout, kind, brilliant Mormon brother (aka in Latter-day Saints circles: "Elder Lindner")—which makes no sense at all, as the highlight of the brunch is all of the adults (Saints excepted), and more than a few of the minors, getting smashed on Tad's wicked-strong sours. The few times we do relent and respect LDS customs, my parents, siblings, in-laws, and I line up outside the teetotaling venue, along the curb, skulking in our cars, gulping the last of our big red Dixie go-cups of vodka, bourbon, or whatever else might lubricate the upcoming experience.

I like alcohol. Too much. More and more, I need less and less of a "reason" to drink. Heavily. Good news, bad news, no news—it doesn't matter.

One afternoon, being that I'm half in the bag on G & Ts, and buoyant, listening to Nat King Cole sing about chestnuts, Rosalie's call finds me receptive. "Merry Christmas," she says.

"And to you." I lift my glass to toast her, telephonically.

"Got another patient for you, if you think you can swing it. I know you're juggling a few, both official ones for us and unofficial ones that you've sort of adopted, like Elmer and Dorothy. I also know it's the holidays, so . . ."

"Which means it's time for giving, no?"

She laughs.

I quaff. "I think I can swing it. Maybe. Give me the rundown."

"Her name is Dolly."

"As in Parton?"

"Yes. Her given name is Gaetana Josephine Ruggieri Graziano."

"My goodness. That explains it."

"Doesn't it??"

Dolly is ninety-four. A widow, she lives with her daughter, Lisa, and son-in-law, Jay, both of whom work full time and have long commutes. "Lisa's very nice but fiercely protective of Dolly." Private, nonhospice nurses visit fifteen hours a day, every day but Sunday. Apparently they come and go at a pretty fast clip, owing to Lisa's high standards of care. Dolly was born in Brooklyn, moved to Vineland, New Jersey, and then Houston. She suffers from advanced heart disease. In fact, her heart's stopped several times. She's a devout Catholic, loves cooking, and hates hospitals. "Lisa says her mother is 'very alert, very with it.' Lisa put in the request but says her mom is totally on board."

"Any special goals . . . like Bob's trip?"

"When I asked this of Lisa, she said her mom has just one goal: stay out of the hospital.

"Maureen Samet is her Haymarket Hospice nurse, Lee Lund her assigned social worker."

## DECEMBER 23, 2009

As I reach for the doorbell, my eyes wander to the unwelcome sign—"No Solicitation"—taped onto the nearest window. It's more than just a sign. My bell-pressing triggers a raucous canine chorus of anti-solicitous yapping.

A black woman opens the front door, invites me in. Dressed in a light greenish-blue blouse and squeaky-soled sneakers, she looks like a nurse to me. "MAUREEN?" I yell. "NICE TO FINALLY MEET YOU."

She shakes her head. "I'm T—"

Tabitha? I wonder. Theresa? Tonya? I just smile and nod, as opposed to asking her to repeat her name. "OH. NICE . . . to meet you. I'm Eric." I try harder to listen.

"Maureen pops by about twice a week. I'm training to be a nurse. I'm here, or someone from my agency is, six days a week while Lisa and Jay are at work. They're here today, but he's running an errand right now. They've been expecting you." She backs up, flush to the wall. "I'll take you to Dolly."

As she escorts me, the racket intensifies. It's crazy loud.

At the end of the foyer, behind one of those collapsible lattice-wood gates, I see two brown dachshunds perched on opposite armrests of the same La-Z-Boy recliner. They're squirming, leaping, yelping, growling, foaming at the mouth—snapping like alligators. They look totally psychotic. Were they pit bulls as opposed to wiener dogs, no way would I continue forward.

"OH!" hollers the nurse-in-training, like a NASA mechanic beside a roaring rocket engine. "THAT'S JUST MOE"—she points left—"AND SLINKY. IGNORE THEM!"

Easier said than done. The pooches are poised for launch. As I inch forward, considering tactics, my fingers skate across my forehead, as if across a Ouija board—probing the scar from ten stitches, courtesy of the Lindner family dog, who seemed a lot less threatening and about the same size as Moe. If they leap at me, do I clock them or haul the nurse-in-training over as a human shield?

But the danger evaporates once the gate's unlocked. The dogs are just excited to see me, not bloodthirsty. Their reddish-brown bodies contort in ecstasy. Tails thump against the La-Z-Boy's corduroy upholstery.

"Moe?" I say. "Slinky?"

Slinky, the larger of the two, hops off the chair and waddles over to retrieve a mangy chew rope.

Dolly giggles. She's a short, tiny thing, even wrapped in a bulky quilt. With her Mediterranean complexion, pretty brown eyes, and neatly arranged gray hair, flecked with black, she could be Golda Meir's (prettier) sister, but for the rosary beads, which she's fingering.

"Dolly," says the quasi-nurse, "this is Eric Lindner."

"Hi, Dolly," I say, walking toward her.

But Moe's not ready to relinquish the limelight. He springs over onto the armrest of Dolly's adjacent La-Z-Boy, inserting himself between the two of us. His wagging tail smacks Dolly on her chin; his tongue shoots out, lapping at me. A jagged, pinkish scar serrates the fur that encases his skull.

"*Moe!*" yells T—. "Get down! Sorry," she says to me. "He's just had brain surgery."

Might wanna ask for your money back.

Dolly smiles, extends her hand, and we clasp. "Hi, Eric," she says. "Get down, Moe. Go play with Slinky." Without a trace of reproof in her voice, she adds, "He's so bad."

"Pull up a chair," says T—.

My left hand still in Dolly's, with my right I grab a chair from the nearby kitchen table, pull it over, and sit. "As I mentioned to your daughter, Lisa, when we spoke over the phone, I just wanted to stop by to introduce myself today, before the holidays. I'm afraid I've got some family commitments for the next couple of weeks, but, come New Year, I'll have more time to visit. I'm really looking forward to it."

"Me, too."

"I've heard such great things about you. You're a superstar."

She lowers her eyes.

"Brought you some cookies and focaccia," I say, holding up a bag.

"Oh . . ."

"Want something to eat, Dolly?" asks T—.

Dolly shakes her head.

"From Red Truck Bakery," I say. "In Warrenton."

Dolly's not let go of my hand. "Such warm hands," she says, squeezing.

The '70s classic *What's My Line?* is on the massive plasma TV. Donning a split-pea soup polyester check suit that includes wide bell bottoms and lapels, host Gene Rayburn is addressing the flamboyantly out-of-the-closet-ahead-of-anyone-else Charles Nelson Reilly, who puffs his pipe and fiddles with his lavender cravat, trying to summon a bon mot.

"I remember that show," I say. "Love those clothes!"

Dolly laughs. It's a lovely sound, innocent and unbridled. It triggers a mini-convulsion. Her head and neck bobble then retract within her collarbone, like a shy Italian turtle.

Once she's regained some composure, with the remote she lowers the volume, and we start getting acquainted. After a while, her daughter ascends from her basement home office and introduces herself. Lisa's got Dolly's tawny complexion and jet-black hair. She and I chat very briefly, then she hustles back downstairs, saying over her shoulder, "I'm afraid I've got to join a conference call, but thank you—so much—for agreeing to visit my mom."

After forty-five minutes, I get set to leave. The first thing I must do is uncouple my hand, which, as Dolly's been gripping it nonstop, by now feels a bit clammy. She's spoken hardly at all . . . but expressed so much, in keeping with Francis of Assisi's advice, "Express love at all times. When necessary, use words."

I lay my free hand atop hers. "I'm sorry my stay this go-round has to be so short, but I'm really looking forward to spending much more time with you as two thousand ten rolls in."

"I hope you have a wonderful Christmas with your family."

"Thank you so much. You too." She releases my hand, I stand, and the dachshunds spring to attention. But their barking and racing about has nothing to do with me. They've heard the garage door open. In walks Jay, Lisa's husband.

We shake hands, get acquainted. While Lisa's energetic and expressive, Jay's stolid and contemplative.

"Bye," I say, waving. "Merry Christmas."

My first report includes the following excerpts:

What a great lady!! Doesn't say much, but she seems sharp as a tack. So pleasant. Daughter says Dolly is almost miraculously better since being pulled from hospital. Good News Story!

## JANUARY 3, 2010

Dolly's such a quiet thing. Though not the same thing as being noncommunicative, it complicates my companionship.

I'm never quite sure how to get the ball rolling. This was never a problem with Bob or Elmer (though it was with Gordon). I never script my visits (with any of my patients), except on those rare occasions when, say, a Haymarket Hospice nurse or a family member asks me to pay particular attention to something or other: the patient's mobility, appetite, mood, etc.

While bounded by the *Dos* and *Don'ts*, every hospice volunteer is encouraged to develop his or her own approach. Mine starts with food. There's something about food. Something atavistic. Once our nasal passages and diaphragms have opened, our taste buds are bubbling, our jaws are chewing, our throats are swallowing, and digestion has begun— we can relax. Once survival is assured, and the hunting and gathering is over (even if the only hunting we do is for a mongo bag of fried pork rinds, the only gathering, two liters of Coke), people open up and can really communicate. With the food doing its work, I like to take a back seat and allow the patient's mind to go wherever they want to take it. For me to act as respondent, a sustainer of whatever they wish to talk about or do, as opposed to my doing the initiating.

I arrive to the same dog show but a different apprentice nurse. I'm armed with more of Red Truck Bakery's famous focaccia, cookies, and muffins. Though I've not got an Italian bone in my body, I've never tasted better bread in my life, so I figure Dolly will flip over it, facilitating our companionship.

I hand her the bag. Her eyes close while the rest of her face brightens as she inhales the aroma of the still-warm bread. "That focaccia you brought last time was the best I've had in years! Maybe ever. Thank you so much!"

I nod toward the loaf. "It's only available on Tuesdays and Fridays, so today's your lucky day."

"Again," says Dolly, as her subtle but unambiguous nod sends the nurse to the kitchen to cut a slice. I explain how this New York City art director relocated from The Big Apple to Orlean, Virginia (home to the smallest Post Office in the country), planted fruit trees, began making jam, then started baking focaccia and pies at home on Friday nights, carting them in the 1954 red Ford farm truck he'd bought from fashion designer Tommy Hilfiger, selling them on an old pine table in a puny but hip general store that was once not so much a filling station, eons ago, as a concrete island with a single pump. "Eventually, he relocates from Sam Drucker's general store, really deep in the boonies, to a defunct Esso service station, across from the old courthouse and gaol, in downtown Warrenton. And, for two years running, the *New York Times* food critic says what this guy pumps out ranks him among the top fifteen food purveyors in the country."

"Standard Oil of New Jersey," says Dolly. "Before Esso, Exxon, ExxonMobil."

"How long'd you live in New Jersey?"

"From the age of six until my late thirties."

The nurse returns with a thick slice of the bread, hands it to Dolly, and says, "Want some water with that?"

"Sure. Thank you." Dolly bites into the crunchy yet spongy focaccia, chews unhurriedly, and swallows. "Oh . . . my . . . God!"

"I'm so glad you like it."

"Want me to cut you a slice, Eric?" asks the nurse, on her way back to the kitchen.

"No, thanks. I can get this any time."

As I conclude the Red Truck story, Dolly seems immersed in a different narrative. The platypus-shaped loaf seems to have transported her somewhere, perhaps back to Brooklyn's Little Italy. One hand clutches her rosary beads, the other, the rosemary-flecked bread. Then her eyes snap open. "Oh, my God! This is so good! It melts in your mouth!"

"Thought you might like it."

"I love it! Such a good Italian bakery, out here . . . But I shouldn't be surprised."

I sense a story. "Why aren't you surprised?"

"I'll tell you why . . . But, first . . ." Beckoning me with her hands, as Italians must learn to do in the womb, she flaps her fingers. "Here . . ." I lean in. She grabs my hands, tugs me, hugs me, and plants a loud, sloppy, olive-oily smooch on my cheek. She holds it for a few seconds, then pulls away, gives my forearms a little shake, releases my hands, and stares into my eyes. "Thank you so much."

"It really is my pleasure."

"So . . . when I get to Houston, in fifty-six, no one's even ever heard of spaghetti! Can you imagine??"

"Hard to. But don't mess with Texas."

She laughs. Her head goes bobble-heady. "I felt so lost. So alone. Like my father, Alexander, when he first arrived in America. But then, thankfully, one day I overhear this woman talking while I'm in line behind her at the A and P. So I say, 'Excuse me, but are you from New Jersey? [*New Joy-zee*]'

"And so she turns around and says to me, 'No, I'm from Brooklyn.'

"'I'm from Brooklyn!' I say."

"That's pretty cool," I interject.

"See, the accents are similar. Brooklyn and Vineland."

"Where's Vineland?"

"Toward the Jersey shore. But not quite there. Moved there from Brooklyn when I was six . . . There, later, when a teenager, my first job was cutting and sewing button-holes at my father's clothing factory. Making button-holes was hard work, and I wasn't too good at it. My fingers were too big." She holds up her hands, introducing them into evidence.

"I like your nails."

"Thank you. The Vietnamese girls added the accents for free. That was so nice. Anyways," she continues, back again in Houston, circa 1956, "so I say to her, 'Know where I can find some spaghetti? All they seem to eat down here is beef and potatoes.'

"'Sure,' she says. And she tells me where there's this great Italian market. After that, we become best friends, her and me. Our husbands too.

"Her husband was a golfing nut. A nut! He was buried with his golf clubs! It made the Texas papers."

"I'll have to tell my dad," I say. "He's a golf fanatic too. I'm sure he'll be quick to change the provisions of his will."

A giggle interrupts Dolly's chewing, sending some food down the wrong pipe. She coughs, reaches for her water, and takes a sip.

But talk of death is dicey, so I backpedal . . . Were Dolly to bring it up—as Elmer often did—I'd be happy to talk of the hereafter.

"My father never played golf," she says. "Not once. That was just for rich Protestants."

"Not just. My dad grew up Catholic. And poor. Worked all day for two bits and six and a half ounces of Coke."

"I can tell your dad's a good person. I miss those cute little Coke bottles."

"My dad's a great person—like you, which I can tell. He's not had a Coke in more than fifty years since working in a bottling plant where he could drink all he wanted and often got sick. But he's as fond of golfing as you are of cooking, from what I understand from Lisa and Rosalie. My father got into golf by caddying *for* rich Protestants up in Syracuse."

"Siracusa!" Her accent sounds perfect (I've been to Sicily). "Many Napolitanos in Syracuse?"

I shrug. "My dad's Polish."

"Oh. Are you Catholic?"

"Well, sort of . . ."

She reaches out and pats my hand. "That's the best we can hope for, Eric. Sort of."

"Got some good Catholic stories, though. Want to hear one?"

She beams, nods, and claps.

"So, years ago, I'm visiting this Polish cathedral with my father, right around the corner from where his father was born, in Warsaw. After stuffing some bills into the brass offering slot, my dad selects a candle, lights it, kneels, and offers up a prayer. Upon rising, he sees me staring at him. He can tell I'm perplexed. 'Why one candle?' he says. I nod. 'For my father,' says he.

"But this perplexes me still more, for if my dad were to make just one offering, I felt for sure he'd make it for my paternal grandmother, Jadwiga, as family lore has it that while Janusz was typically off gallivanting with his vodka-guzzling ex-pat pals . . . when, that is, not globetrotting with some nubile maiden he'd picked up in Milwaukee, Detroit, or Chicago, while—ostensibly—peddling Krakus hams (he was a franchisee), pushing Polish Bonds (he was a broker), gathering intel for the CIA (he was a suspected spy), or lobbying for his pet project, the U.S. Congress's commemorating in 1964 the millennial anniversary of Poland's founding (he was a fierce patriot, but also saw the opportunity for some nice profits, via the sale of medals)—his dutiful, faithful workhorse wife was at home raising four boys while keeping the large-circulation Polish newspaper press cleaned, oiled, and humming."

Dolly's eye roll suggests intimate familiarity with this sort of division of labor.

"So I give voice to my confusion: 'Dad, why not your mother?'"

"My dad smiles. 'My saintly mother doesn't need a candle.'"

Dolly slaps her palms against her cheeks, making *The Scream* face, Naples style.

"I know I've not known you long, Dolly, but I'm a fairly quick study and a good judge of character. For instance, I proposed to the most amazing woman in the world after just six dates."

"Oh! What's her name?"

"Ellen. We've been married almost twenty-four years."

She pats my hand then squeezes. "Good . . . good!"

"My judgment is this: no one will ever need to light a candle for you, either."

She bats her eyes then pulls me in for a smooch. "My father's family lived not far from Bari, on a tiny island, off the tip of Italy's boot—" But then a shroud of reverent sadness falls upon her, like a malfunctioning curtain call. She shakes her head, covering her face with her hands. "Oh . . ."

I sense a wider window into her lovely character. More important, I sense a connection, a way to enhance my role as a companion.

But I also see the warning sign: visible emotion, in her tone of voice and body language. Rosalie taught me that getting too personal—unless the patient takes the lead—can be hazardous.

Given terminally ill patients' (understandably) emotionally fraught state, it can even be problematic when they invite questions. Questions lead to questions and to memories, not all of which are happy. I'm not sure if this is a place to charge ahead—or fall back.

I opt for the former. "Can you tell me a little about your dad?"

"Know what the first words Papa said when he laid eyes on my mama?"

"What?"

Though her shoulders and hands do most of the communicating, Dolly does say, "Mama mia!"

"For real?"

She nods. "But Papa—Alexander—wasn't ready to meet Mama, being all grimy in his work clothes . . . seeing her as he looked up from his sewing machine, along Atlantic City's boardwalk. So elegant was Mama, and so well protected, too! Flanked by her Napolitano family!"

"What a great image! Must've been hard for him to keep his seams straight!"

She claps, laughs, then points at me, excitedly. "You understand, don't you?"

"Well, if it's love at first sight you're talking about, well then, yes, I do understand. I was stricken the first time I laid eyes on my bride-to-be, too."

"I want to hear!"

"First I want to hear more of your story."

Dolly's tone rises and falls several octaves, her hands are a gesticulated blur, her torso rocks forward and back . . . "After saying, 'Mama mia!' Papa says to his coworker, 'I a-see-a the woman I'm a-gonna marry!'"

Suddenly her body grows still. "Then, when in Maine, in Kennebunkport, where he sang each summer with a troupe from Brooklyn, Papa dies. Of a massive heart attack. He was with Mama—looking at her, as he always did . . . while singing his favorite verse to his favorite song: 'Let me call you sweetheart, I'm in love with you . . .'" Dolly's head droops.

## FEBRUARY 22

I detect some disturbing trends. More oxygen. More blacking out on the toilet. From just taking pills for her heart to wearing a nitroglycerine patch. Visible fatigue; admitting to "feeling blue" and "worried." For nearly three hours, Dolly hardly says a word. We just sit, hold hands, and channel surf between the Olympics and her favorite game shows. Yet, still, when asked how she's doing, her typical reply is as follows, as excerpted from my report:

"Doing okay. Pretty good. I thank God for every day."

## MARCH 8

I get a frantic call, seeing if I can visit Dolly. As I walk in, she removes her oxygen mask.

Intercepting me and pulling me aside, the nurse whispers how it all started with a panic attack. It kept Dolly from getting a manicure, so I know it was serious.

Dolly and I talk about going on an outing, to an Italian restaurant. But we both sense she's not up to it. After an hour or so she nods off, and I head off.

## MAY 7

Dolly and I are watching more and more TV, especially *The Ellen De-Generes Show*, *Everybody Loves Raymond*, and various game shows, both old and new. During Ellen's 2010 Mother's Day special, when the Guest Dancer of the Day appears on stage to shake her booty before the yip-yipping studio audience—her acrobatic gyrating, air-humping, and big-belly rubbing just this side of pornographic—the crowd goes nuts, as do Dolly and I. When Dolly starts gasping for air, I glance around to make sure the oxygen tank is nearby.

The laughter brings respite. But not much. Dolly's having more problems, day and night. She's not reporting this to me but to her nurses, who relay it to me. Like several other patients, Dolly is intent on keeping as much bad news from me as possible, as if it's her job to be a jolly companion, as if she's worried that were I to really know the gravity of her situation I'd bolt.

But Dolly's no Meryl Streep. She may be able to suppress her voice, but much as she'd like she can't control her nonverbal communication. I feel the worry in her firmer grip . . . see it in her wandering eyes . . . infer it from her calling Jay home from work (Lisa's drive is too long), which exacerbates selfless Dolly's sadness . . . in inconveniencing her kind son-in-law.

## MAY 28

I've been really busy, traveling a lot, juggling a host of family and work-related issues. But Dolly wants to see me, so I make time. My report captures where things stand.

> Noteworthy "event" . . . HH [Haymarket Hospice] alerted. Lisa asked me to come over. Dolly . . . more fatigued. Had another A.M. "pinching/ pressure"—received meds.

The next day, I ring Lisa. "How's your mom doing?"

"Better. But we're worried. Thank you so much for coming by. It eases her panic attacks."

"Whenever I'm able, you can count on me. I can't guarantee I *can* come, but you should *never* feel shy about calling me."

"Thank you so much."

"Any idea what might have triggered the panic attack?"

"Lots of things could have. She's just had it so rough for so long. Life's really been hard on her . . ."

"So often," I say, "it seems the sweetest people carry the heaviest burdens."

"That sums up my mom's situation . . . The way her dad died . . ."

"She told me the story. So sad, and poignant."

"She tell you about her son, my brother . . . and her husband, my dad?"

"No."

"Got a minute?"

"Sure."

Lisa tells me how first Dolly's son then her husband die—almost back to back. The former in a freak accident, in Bali, the latter when blood clot formed after a fall in Texas just as the two were about to settle on a new place and a new life of relaxed retirement. "Know what she said to me, Eric?"

"Huh?"

"'Leo Junior's dying made a hole in my heart.' Then, when my dad dies, 'Now I've got two holes in my heart.' Mom never really recovered after Dad died."

"I am so, so sorry, Lisa."

"And now, with her own health? She hates being a burden and wants to contribute. For longer than she should have, she insisted on driving, shopping, cooking, taking care of Moe and Slinky, helping out around the house. But now she can't even leave the house any more. She can't hardly leave her La-Z-Boy other than to go to the toilet or bed. Her immobility and disability get her so depressed . . . like she's not doing her share . . ."

"How hard it must be for your mom. For someone—'course I've not known her long at all—who seems so enthusiastic, and energetic."

"That's Mom alright."

"And how hard it must be for you, too."

"We love having her around. She's an inspiration. I just wish I could be around more often. That work wasn't so demanding . . . such a long commute."

"Well, I'm just thankful I can help out, a little. Whenever I visit with her, she's all smiles, compliments, hugs, and happiness. Always asking about my day. Wanting to hear that I've got no worries in my life. Your mom's amazing."

"Thank you. She really is."

## JULY 20

I'm feeling guilty. I shouldn't, but I am. Dolly's heading downhill just as I'm heading out of the country twenty-six out of the next thirty-one days. "It's the worst stretch I've had," Dolly manages to tell me during a bout of crying (and my own bout, fighting the urge to cry). She's passing out more and more on the toilet. She's bolting upright at night, terrified. The pinching pressure in her chest now presents as much during the day as it has been at night. She's taking more medication, but while it may be helping her heart it's giving her "terrible headaches." For the past month, each time I've arrived she's looked a little more tired, a little more drained, a little more defeated.

Trying to abide by the *Do* of keeping the entire Haymarket Hospice team in the loop, I send Rosalie an e-mail, asking her to inform Maureen, Lee, and everyone else of my travels.

## JULY 26

I manage to squeeze in a visit just prior to heading out for dinner with Ellen to celebrate our twenty-fourth wedding anniversary. Soon after I arrive, Maureen Samet shows up. As it's our first time meeting face to face, we take a moment to get better acquainted. She appears to be in her early forties, solidly built like those old black-and-white photos of pioneering Oregon Trail women, maybe 5'8", with medium-length chestnut hair. Her attire is half registered nurse, half rural Clarke County, a lovely part of Northern Virginia. While Maureen's as easygoing in person as over the phone, she's all business, too, wasting no time firing up her laptop and taking vitals. "I heard you had a bad night, Dolly," she says.

"I'm better now."

"The nitro worked, then? You were able to fall back to sleep?"

"Uh-huh."

"On a scale of one to ten, before taking the pill, how'd you describe the intensity of the pain, with one being lowest, ten the highest?"

"About a three or four."

"I mean before taking the pill."

"Oh."

I interject, "Tell the truth, Dolly."

She blinks. "Four or five."

Maureen shakes her head while tapping the laptop keys. "And after?"

"One, maybe?" Dolly changes the subject. "Have some of Eric's cookies, Maureen."

"There'll be time for that, Dolly," I say.

Maureen eyes me, thankful that we're on the same page. "First the checkup, then the victuals." Maureen's got a lovely schtick she uses to distract her patients from the seriousness of their condition, and she employs it brilliantly here. While with her stethoscope listens to Dolly's chest, Maureen says, "You heard the expression, 'Does a bear shit in the woods?'"

Never do I ever hear Dolly cuss, but she sure enjoys a good, "earthy" tale. Maureen's the Mother Earth of such tales. So accustomed is she to Maureen's yarns, even before the nurse begins spooling hers out, Dolly starts clapping and giggling, causing her head to bobble, the La-Z-Boy to squeak.

"Well, let me tell you," Maureen says, while continuing to listen and tap away, "not only do bears shit in the woods, but their turds are gi-NOR-mous!"

"Oh, my God!" Dolly's bobble head retracts deep into her collarbone.

"So, last week," says Maureen, "I'm in the kitchen, and outside on my front porch I hear this racket. So I look out the window, and, lo and behold, there's this bear. A big, fat thing, and he's just sitting on his haunches—eating one of my cooling pies! Like Winnie-the-Pooh eating all that honey?? The sucker'd snatched it off my windowsill! I'm so mad!"

"Oh, my God!" exclaims Dolly.

"What kind of pie, Maureen?" I ask.

"Cherry."

Clap. "Yum! Oh, my God!"

Maureen's voice drops, in keeping with the gravity of the crime: "You know how long it takes to pit the cherries needed for just one pie?? More than an a hour, just to do the pitting, let alone the crust, which I make from scratch. And this greedy bear's scarfing my pie in a matter of seconds! So I rap on the window. 'Hey!' I yell. 'Put down that pie, and scat!'"

By this time, Dolly and I are both in stitches. We're tapping each other on the arm, pointing at Maureen like we've got the best seat in the house at the best comedy club in America.

But I challenge Maureen. "Are you making this up?"

"I am not," she insists, "as God is my witness!"

"Oh, my God!" mutters the devout Dolly, before crossing herself.

"Finally, after screaming as loud as I can and banging pots and pans, the bear drops the empty, mangled pie plate, gets up, and saunters off my porch. Not like he's in any sort of hurry, mind you. For he's finished eating. Finished doing something else, too. For when I go out onto the porch, to clean up the mess, what do I find? That pig of a bear's done left me a present! A *huuuuge* crap!"

A spasm of laughter propels Dolly's torso forward, further than I've ever seen her in the Lay-Z-Boy. "Oh, my God, Maureen! No!"

"As God is my witness, Dolly. And when I say huge, I do mean *huuuuge*! It was so big, and because I knew people might not believe me, I took a photo of it. I even laid it against a piece of paper, eight and a half by eleven inches, to put it into perspective." She fiddles with her cell phone, retrieving some digital evidence of the pilfering bear's prodigious defecation.

Dolly takes a peek then turns away. "Oh, my God!" Her entire body is shaking now, like she's sitting atop the epicenter of a La-Z-Boy earthquake. The recliner is squeaking like mad.

Once Maureen leaves, perhaps because it's my wedding anniversary, Dolly and I get onto the topic of her nuptials. She waxes nostalgic about her cake. "It was so beautiful! I can still see them unloading it—so carefully—from the back of a van. Fer-something . . . the baker's name. They drove—so slowly—over the Brooklyn Bridge. Not only was it so pretty, but how it tasted!" In the Italian way, she pincers her fingers, brings them to her mouth, then explodes them away, exclaiming "Mmm-waaaa!"

"You're making me hungry!"

"It wasn't just the wedding cake. Their pignoli?? Oh, my God!"

"Pignoli?"

"Pine nut cookies. I've never seen them anywhere else. Not since my wedding."

A few days later, while out of town, I surf the Internet and track down Ferraro's in Manhattan's Little Italy. According to its website, it's "America's first espresso bar." I give some thought to ordering Dolly a wedding cake, the sort of buttercream fantasy she'd had on her big day, back in the '30s. But this would have required some tricky logistics, as, in order to maintain quality control, Ferraro's doesn't deliver outside the five Boroughs. So I zero in on what can safely and reliably be baked in Little Italy and delivered to Virginia's Piedmont: the pignoli. I wish I could have been there when the food arrived. I smile at the thought of her learning she's got a "big delivery," opening the boxes, and being transported back to happier times.

## AUGUST 12

As I enter the house, I sense something's wrong. First, the front door's unlocked. It's never unlocked. Second, Dolly's not in her La-Z-Boy. I've never seen her anywhere but in her living room recliner. (Or returning to it from the bathroom.) Third, the dogs are subdued. A few initial yaps, but none with feeling. They look drugged.

It's a new nurse. Not from Haymarket Hospice. She introduces herself. "I'll take you to her. She's in her bedroom."

During the course of nine months and forty-three visits, I've never even seen Dolly's bedroom, let alone entered it. The Holy of Holies.

Just before we enter, glancing at the bakery bags I'm holding, the nurse pulls me aside. "She doesn't have an appetite."

We'll see.

"She's talked a lot about you. She's so glad to see you."

"Same here."

"She was worried she might not ever see you . . . again. Oh, and she's embarrassed about how she looks."

"How she looks? What do you mean?"

"Oh, she doesn't look bad at all. She's just, you know, not up to her usual self. Hair's not made up. She's still in her nightclothes. That sort of thing."

"Oh." Dolly's never been the least bit vain. She's just like my mom and dad: old school. Proper attire and grooming an expression of civility and politeness, not vanity. So Dolly always wants her hair brushed, her gown neat, her nails at least trimmed.

I enter her bedroom to the sound of Howie Mandel badgering some poor contestant on *Deal or No Deal?* Dolly's quarters are half suburban bedroom, half hospital room: a vintage chest of drawers vies with the sort of gray, state-of-the-art bed typical of 5,300 other American hospices; a mahogany cabinet fights for space with an articulated rolling tray table, on which sits an orange plastic cup with a neon-green bendy straw and a tray of uneaten (seemingly untouched) food.

Dolly looks really depressed. The gravity of her bad deal is clearly weighing on her.

"Oh, Eric! I'm so glad you're here!" She throws out her hands, struggling not to cry.

I'm struggling harder, I think. She appears so frail and finally—or nearly—defeated.

"I was wor—" Her voice breaks.

I rest my hand on her shoulder.

"Worried that I wouldn't see you again."

A lump forms in my throat, joining the knot in my stomach.

She clutches my hand. "Such warm hands."

Hers are cold. "Warm from your heart, Dolly." I locate the remote and mute Mandel.

"I must look terrible," she says.

"Mission impossible. You look beautiful." I mean it, too. The most beautiful images I've ever seen are not the stunning creations painted by Van Gogh or Vermeer but the sublimely transfixing photos of a supernova's demise, snapped by Hubble.

My supernova squeezes my hands, then withdraws one of hers to dab a tear. "Oh . . ."

"I hear you've had a rough go of it. I'm really sorry I wasn't around to be with you."

She squeezes harder.

"You get my postcard, at least?"

She nods toward her tray table, where the postcard of Old Town Warsaw leans against a lamp. "I've missed you so much. Seeing you is the highlight of my week."

"You're my highlight, Dolly. How you doing right now?"

"I'm okay," she lies. "I thank God for every day. Every day is a blessing."

"That's the spirit. I know I'm certainly blessed, knowing you."

She starts sobbing. "They . . . won't even let me . . . get out of bed!"

"You feel you can? Want to?"

She nods, but her tone of voice is a reality check. "I was in the hospital for a few days. Passed out at home again. They didn't think I'd . . ." She diverts her eyes to the wall.

Now it's my turn to do the hand squeezing.

"Poor Lisa and Jay," she says. "They're worried about their vacation. They've not had a vacation for years."

"Stop worrying, Dolly."

"That's what Jay said, too. 'Don't worry.'"

"Trust me, Dolly, you truly have nothing to worry about, whether you and I see each other many more times on this round rock we now inhabit or very few. There's a room prepared for you—elsewhere. Upstairs. For sure. I'm as sure of it as I've been of anything in my life. And you know who the caterer is upstairs, right?"

She shakes her head.

"Ferraro's."

"Oh! I forgot to thank you!" Tears stream down her cheeks in thin, jerky rivulets.

"Brought you something else."

She's attentive, wicking away her tears with the back of her free hand. "Some cake."

"Oh, no!"

"From Heidelberg. Want me to cut you a slice or two?"

"Two?"

"Two cakes today. Chocolate and lemon."

"Oh, my God!"

"I asked Elle, 'What's your best cake today?' And she said 'Chocolate or lemon.' So, naturally, I had to get both. For my girl. You know my motto: When it comes to food, if you don't have to choose, why choose?"

"Oh, my God! I'll have a slice of each." She pats my hand then wags her finger. "Not too big, though. Got to watch my figure."

I step outside Dolly's room and wave at the nurse. "Could you please bring Dolly a slice from each cake?"

She looks shocked. "You got her to agree to eat??"

I nod. "We got history."

When the nurse returns after a few minutes, she's yet to cut the cakes. They're still in their boxes. "I've got to show you the cakes first, Dolly. Aren't they're pretty??"

"Oh!"

"I'll be right back," says the nurse. "For you, too, Eric?"

"No, thanks."

When her cakes arrive, Dolly first turns to the chocolate. She doesn't wolf it. Like Bob Zimmerman with his pancakes, she's methodical. Pondering and calibrating how much to hive off with her fork. Steering the portion carefully to her mouth. Snagging dollops of errant icing with her tongue. Chewing slowly. Prolonging the enjoyment.

"Elle's a good German," I say, "and she makes a darned good German cake. She doesn't cut corners. You know Germans!"

"Hah!" Some dark crumbs tumble from her mouth. I tidy her up by patting her chin and lips with a napkin, grab her soda from the tray table, and arrange the bendy straw. She sips, swallows. "You can tell it's from scratch," she says. "Fresh. It makes such a big difference."

I return her drink to the table. "Germans . . . they don't mess around."

"I know! My neighbor in Houston was German. She kept her kitchen spotless. It always embarrassed me."

"Well, Germans have their strengths and their weaknesses, too. They make great cars and tanks, but they can't make meatballs with Sunday sauce like you!"

"No, they can't! They're not big on tomatoes, are they?"

"Come to think of it, no, they're not."

"Oh, how I loved to cook! How I miss it so!"

After we talk a bit more, I say, "I really hate having to leave, but I've got a flight to catch." Dolly pulls me in for a send-off hug and an especially long, loud, sloppy smooch.

Out of nowhere, Maureen appears, shaking her head in mock disapproval. "Get a room! Listen . . . can you lend me a hand? Got a few minutes? Not in a hurry, are you?"

"Eric's on his way to the air—" Dolly begins before my head shaking silences her.

"I got some time, Maureen," I lie, fretting about making my flight. I obsessed about getting to the airport early even before 9/11, even before my titanium hip implants and hefty bag full of eye drops on account of my cornea implant necessitated that far more time be allotted.

"Great," says Maureen as she pops open her laptop and fires it up.

Meanwhile, Dolly and I communicate nonverbally. She's worried I'll miss my flight.

Perceptively noticing the beads of sweat on Dolly's forehead, Maureen directs me to help her remove the heavy quilt and adjust Dolly's body so she's more comfortable. "There now," says Maureen. "That better?"

Dolly nods. "Much. Thank you."

Maureen frowns, playfully. "If you're not comfortable, Dolly, you've got to tell someone."

"Okay."

Maureen asks, "Wanna try and get up and walk?"

"Okay."

"Feel up to it?"

Dolly nods.

Employing the walker and other props, Maureen and I slowly, carefully hoist Dolly up onto the edge of the bed. "'Kay," says Maureen, as she steps back a few inches, like one does when their child first pedals off without the aid of training wheels.

Dolly doesn't move. She flails about, trying to latch onto something, finally clasping the bed-frame. Her feet dangle, toes inches from the floor. With a discreet head tilt, Maureen directs my eyes to Dolly's lips. They're purple-blue from exertion and fear.

Seeing her frozen so makes me think of that poignant point of pure, cold honesty, when a patient knows or—perhaps worse—when suspicion first dawns on denial's horizon—that any further attempt to eke out more Time is preordained to fail. How unforgiving must it be, that solitary moment of bracing consciousness, when "terminal" eclipses "ill" . . . freighted with the foreboding comprehension that there shall be no more mini-remissions or plateauing of symptoms . . .

Bob Zimmerman drifts into Dolly's room, seated in his chair. He waves at me, smiles, then begins trying to hoist himself up . . .

Ellen Hensley and Gordon Ford float in . . . like Dolly, in their beds . . . and resume struggling . . . *It's okay*, I whisper telepathically to them. *You can stop now . . . You can let go.*

It's as if Dolly hears me. She stares at the floor . . .

Would it be easier if were Dolly "out of it," mentally? Was it easier for Ellen, given her Alzheimer's? Or Bob, given his? Christianity, Buddhism, Jungian theory, etc., etc., say denial is irrational, sinful, unconscious.

But is it? Always? Mightn't it not instead be, at the End, the apex of rationality, sinlessness, and consciousness? Just because we "know" certain things we love will end . . . that certain people we adore—we'll not again see—must we embrace such knowledge?

And what is knowledge, exactly? What ends? What begins? Certainly the Hasidim had a peculiar take on things . . . dancing—by all accounts joyously—while awaiting their turn in the Zyklon B showers . . . as others rent whatever scraps they were wearing, sobbed, blubbered, or swelled with fury . . . finding the irrational reaction of their Eastern brethren even more incomprehensible than the cool rationality of Nazi evil.

"Just sit there a bit, Dolly," says Maureen. "Get your bearings. Catch your breath. Don't push yourself."

Dolly shakes her head. "I want to lie back down."

"That's totally fine," says Maureen. She and I help Dolly back onto her bed. Using the control pad, Maureen adjusts the settings to make things more comfortable. "That about right?"

Dolly's nod is listless, limp. She's too wrecked—and dejected—to say a word or even summon her natural smile.

"I'll write you from Poland," I say.

Maureen taps my forearm. "I'll head into the kitchen so you lovebirds can say good-bye."

Dolly rallies, finds her voice: "Make sure to have some of the cake Eric brought."

"Oh, I will! Don't you worry! Eric and his food! His vicarious gluttony is famous!"

Once Maureen's gone, Dolly pulls me close. Forcefully, with both hands. All of a sudden she's got Popeye forearms. "I love you so much, Eric!"

## AUGUST 19

I'm six thousand miles away, on business, walking along the Baltic coast with my country manager, just east of Gdańsk. I'm thinking about Dolly because I've just bought her a postcard and she'd love it here at this time of year, as the place is so festive during the three-week-long celebration of St. Dominic, one of her favorite saints. Wanting her to receive the postcard before I'm back home, I'm thinking about where to buy a stamp, when and where to mail it . . . My cell phone rings. The number's blocked. "Hello?"

"Eric?"

"Yes. Hi, Jay."

"I'm afraid Dolly's passed. The good news is she went quietly. She didn't experience any pain. We thought you'd want to know. And we wanted to thank you."

That night I drink so much vodka even the Poles take notice. (That's saying something.) I can't stop thinking about why so many lovely people must suffer so.

It's not a quantitative thing. Dolly lived ninety-four years, fifteen years longer than her 1915 cohort.

It's a qualitative thing. If there were such a market, a new "Pit" in Chicago, say, where one could effect trades in such things, would

Dolly have swapped a decade—for another weekend with her father? No question. And how about her sweet Leonardo Jr.? Or her lovely husband, who'd worked so hard to be able to enjoy his retirement with Dolly—and she, with him—only to die before being able to reap a second of what he'd so conscientiously sown? How many decades would Dolly have swapped for each year—or week or day or minute or second or solitary heartbeat—with her loved ones who'd predeceased her?

Or even . . . not just to be with them but to allow them to live instead of her. Yes, Dolly would've traded her time for theirs. You ask me, University of Chicago cosmologists and Princeton University philosophers would do well to fret less about whether the Universe flared forth 13.714159 billion years ago, so as to be able to redeploy some of their prodigious intellects to fathoming Dolly's supernova sense of time. You ask me, the Catholic Church's 204 mystery-loving cardinals need to join hands with science's 1,500 string theorists feverishly scribbling mystifying mathematical formulae regarding what even they admit they'll never see, let alone understand, and together have a look at the manifest simplicity of what tugged Dolly's heartstrings.

My country manager is as grounded in irony as they come. During the height of the Cold War, his father, an anti-Commie engineer, worked at the mammoth Ursus tractor factory (the world's largest) where, in the event the Politburo gave the green light, he was to throw a lever and switch over from making tractors—to tanks. Now this child of the Warsaw Pact is a friend of and owes his livelihood to a child of NATO. As my manager has seen more than his fair share of silent, drunken brooding, he leaves me alone. He understands that talking isn't essential to communicating. He knows that, sometimes, it's best to let what's inside stay inside.

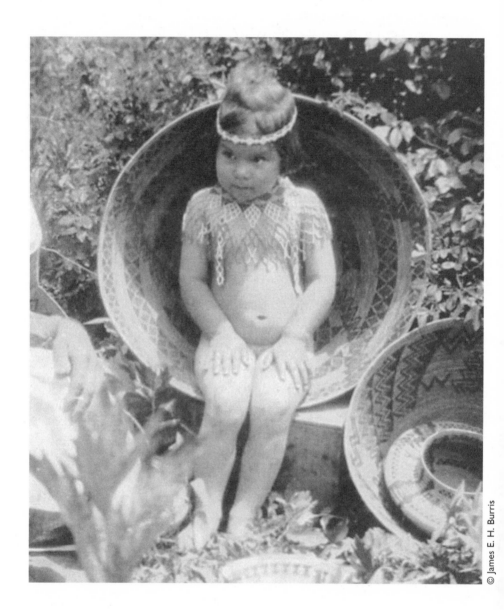

# WE'RE ONLY AS SICK
# AS OUR SECRETS

**O**ver the course of nine months, despite the passing of eight very special people, the joy of hospice has outweighed the sadness. Alfred Lord Tennyson was right: "'Tis better to have loved and lost than never to have loved at all."

That said, though my hospice is fulfilling, it is encroaching on my ability to provide companionship for my own parents. It's also getting in the way of my spending as much time as I'd like with my wife. I still have two kids, still run a company based in Poland. Consequently, when Rosalie calls and asks if I'd be willing to take on another assignment, I hesitate. Counting both official (Dolly's as ebullient as ever at this point in time) and unofficial (Elmer's chopping as much wood as ever) patients, my current roster stands at five.

However, Rosalie is an amazing, compassionate advocate, and cagey, too. She hooks my conscience and preempts my objections by noting—right off—that this new patient lives very close to me. "She'd be, by far, the closest you've had. You could just pop by from time to time while you're out and about and you've got a few minutes."

"You win. Give me the scoop."

Like Dolly, Mary Louise Burris is ninety-four. She was born November 5, 1915, on a Mono Reservation, just south of North Fork,

California, east of Yosemite. Her father was Irish, her mother, 50 percent Native American. Mary Louise's first job was cleaning up after the rough crowd that patronized her aunt's boardinghouse, but she studied at night, worked hard, and ended up in a highly classified position with Strategic Air Command during the Cold War, where she was the gatekeeper through whom papers and packages intended for the top brass had to pass. She retired in the early '80s. She's been widowed, twice, and lives alone. With her husband, Charles, and her only child, Jim Burris, she moved to Maryland from California. When Jim relocated to Northern Virginia, he arranged for her to move five miles northeast of me.

I ask, "Who called you guys requesting a companion?"

"Jim," says Rosalie.

"Is Mary Louise on board?"

"I'm not sure, to be honest. She's very upset at the moment. Her best friend just died—Jim's mother-in-law. I'm told this death came totally unexpected. Also, apparently, it's served to aggravate what was already a strained relationship between Jim and Mary Louise."

"How strained?"

"Not sure." Mary Louise's medical problems range from early Alzheimer's to advanced congestive heart disease, like Gordon Ford. Also like Gordon, Mary Louise is on a respirator, "but she's much more ambulatory. She uses oxygen a fair bit and is allowed—that's odd—oxycodone every hour."

"What's odd?"

"The hourly part."

"Why?"

"It's strong. Hourly doses are more typical with, say, bone cancer, given how painful it is. Not so much with congestive heart disease."

"How's it administered?"

"Ampules."

"Ampules?"

"It's a small delivery device that facilitates portion control. Plastic or glass, it's filled from a bottle, via a syringe.

"How long has Mary Louise got, you think, in your opinion? Weeks? Months?"

"I'd rather not speculate." Mary Louise lives at The Oaks, an independent-living complex across the street from Oak Springs, a "skilled-nursing facility" to which The Oaks residents can avail themselves on an à la carte basis. She doesn't procure any such assistance but does spend considerable time enjoying her brand-new plasma TV, which, just before dying, Jim's mother-in-law bought her. "Apparently, it was a gift given for no other reason but simple friendship. I mean, it wasn't an early birthday present, a late Christmas present, et cetera." Mary Louise especially loves watching sports: football, baseball, and ice hockey.

"Anything special she'd like to do?"

"Now that you ask, yes. Of utmost importance to her is writing some sort of letter to her granddaughter. Maymie is her only grandchild. Jim hopes you can help his mother complete it. I'm not sure of the nature of the letter."

"Well, I'll certainly try. I'll call Mary Louise tomorrow."

"Great. Thank you so much. But I need to warn you . . ."

"Yes?"

"Based on what I've heard, and the reports I've reviewed, Mary Louise is very picky—and prickly. She rejected my previous volunteer."

"Has she agreed to my visiting?"

"Not exactly."

## MARCH 30, 2010

"Hel-lo?"

"Is this Mrs. Burris?"

"It is. With whom am I speaking?" Her gravelly voice seems cordial but discriminating.

"My name's Eric Lindner. I understand that Rosalie Palermo spoke with you? Told you I'd call?"

"She did."

"Well, I'm just calling to see if, and when, I might pop by to introduce myself."

"Now's not a good time, I'm afraid."

"Okay."

"My best friend just died. My daughter-in-law's mother, no less."

"Rosalie told me. I'm so very sorry."

"Thank you. The funeral is next week. Things are a bit hectic right now."

"I can only imagine. I hope things go as well as, well, possible. I'll ring you toward the end of next week."

I ring her six days later. "Now's still not a good time," she says.

I ring her three days after that. "Sorry. Not a good time . . ."

I'm getting the sense she thinks it'll never be a good time. But I don't take it personally.

It's often hard persuading patients to allow companions into their lives. The family might want it. Friends might say it's a great idea. A chorus of professionals might sing the hallelujahs of hospice care. But none of this matters. It all boils down to whether a patient wants a stranger entering his or her life. There are few remaining opportunities to influence the course of her life, and it's the patient's prerogative to allow in—or to exclude—whomever, whenever.

It's seldom a matter of cost. Most hospice services are covered by Medicare or are otherwise free of charge. As we approach the End, money's just about irrelevant. What's relevant is preserving a shred of privacy and dignity, which can be tough when you're incontinent, your wig's on backward, or you can't find your false teeth.

Few are like Bob Zimmerman, who'd incessantly pestered Rosalie, seeking a companion. Most are, instead, nervous, cautious, skeptical, embarrassed, ambivalent, or all of the above. Some are completely against an alien intruder materializing out of nowhere just as they're making their final arrangements—like that high-powered D.C. attorney with pancreatic cancer and Indian immigrant with AIDS who wanted nothing whatsoever to do with me.

That Mary Louise's son, Jim, wants me to visit hardly seals the deal. If anything, based on what Rosalie's told me, it may have only made matters worse, what with mother and son at odds, for whatever reason.

I've found this often to be the case, unfortunately: the lack of a meeting of the minds. You'd think there'd be an overwhelming desire by loved ones—to converge. You'd think that, this being the last chance for, say, a parent and a child to make peace—they'd jump at it. But instead, sadly, far too often some silly new skirmish rekindles a long-simmering dispute, based on some hoary injury or insult, decades old, often imagined. Instead of the End acting as a softening agent, it often adds more crust to the scab.

I'm not sure how raw things are between Jim and Mary Louise. Maybe things have been blown out of proportion. Perhaps I'll learn more, but perhaps I won't.

Maybe she's decided that she knows best, determining that she doesn't need me, or want me. She certainly seems very independent, living alone and all. Though I've yet to meet her, and we've only spoken a bit, she seems with it, mentally. Maybe she's settled into a quasi-comfortable routine and, to her way of seeing things—the only viewpoint that matters—injecting someone new into her ninety-fifth year involves undue risk.

But as an attorney and businessman, much of my professional career has involved figuring out how to ameliorate risk. I can also be a fairly decent salesman. Being a lawyer helps. I'm well trained in the art of prostitution. Adept at making risk molehills seem mountainous, I've successfully whored myself out to many a corporate and governmental client in the United States and Europe by concocting some sort of risk-reducing "value-added."

"Years ago," I say to Mary Louise, "I helped a preeminent legal scholar organize and edit his work. I'd love to see if I can help you in a similar fashion."

"And what was this scholar's field of expertise?"

"Insanity law."

"Well, then, I'm sure we'll get along fine. I'm delighted you called."

"When might I stop by?"

"Call back next week, maybe."

"I will. I'm really looking forward to meeting you, Mrs. Burris."

It's not until my fourth call that our chat runs beyond a few minutes. She does most of the talking.

"These days, my goal is to stay sane. A tall order. I can hardly see my own two feet, what with my macular degeneration."

"My dad has that, too. It's hard."

"I've just cracked a tooth . . . Hurts like heck. Got gout. The so-called rich white man's disease. But I'm not rich, white, or male. I'm a half-breed Mono Indian. Quarter-breed, to be precise. Maybe you'll see my papoose."

"I'd really like that."

"Hanging right behind me, above my head. Darn shingles!"

As I listen to her scratching, she asks, "Ever had shingles?"

"Yes. Very painful. But they went away as quickly as they'd come, thankfully."

"Lucky you. Mine's scorched across my head. It feels like my hair's on fire. My ear burns, drives me crazy. I want to scratch my scalp off. Hah! Get the pun?"

I get it, but I'm not sure what to say. She's thrown so much at me, so quickly.

"I get panic attacks, too," she continues. Her laundry list of maladies doesn't even include her main problem: congestive heart failure. "You sure you're up for this assignment?"

"We'll see, Mrs. Burris. We'll see."

"That we shall. So, listen, maybe you can help me? . . ."

"I hope so."

"My doctor just yanked my Xanax. Can't understand why. Been taking the stuff for years. Panic attacks. Never had a problem. I don't pop the things like gumdrops."

"I'll look into it, Mrs. Burris."

"Thank you. So, shall we schedule a visit?"

"Let's." Yeah! I'm not sure why she's relented. Maybe I sound like an ally, as regards her medication. Maybe the loss of her best friend has had a chance to sink in and the absence of companionship is now more keenly felt. Maybe . . . any number of reasons.


## APRIL 13


I arrive at The Oaks, take the elevator to the second floor, and wend my way around to her apartment. The door's ajar. "Hello?" I inquire.

"Come on in." I enter. May Louise is directly in front of me, in the far corner of her small unit, seated in an easy chair, dressed in the sort of loose-fitting floral gown my folks wear when they're in the hospital. Behind her, on the wall, is the wicker papoose in which she was carted when a tribal baby in central California. A big TV is tuned to a Washington Nationals baseball game. A ventilator is affixed to her face, its tubing connected to a wheeled oxygen tank parked on the floor by her feet. Her breathing is labored, her skin is the color of the McDonald's mocha frappé I bring another of my patients, and her salt-and-pepper hair is short, in a bun. She's wearing glasses.

"Hello," I say, extending my hand. She shakes it. I hold up a tin of coconut patties purchased at the West Palm airport. "Just got back from seeing my parents. My dad's eighty-three. My mom's eighty-four. She likes younger men."

She removes the ventilator. "I do, too. But I don't like coconut." Returning the oxygen-delivery contraption to her face, she motions for me to take a seat on the adjacent sofa.

"Sorry!" I sit.

"You didn't know," she says out of one side of her mask.

"I grew up with the Senators. They move to Texas, then they start playing decent ball."

She rips off her mask—like a catcher after a foul ball. "I follow the Caps, too. But especially the Redskins."

I've got such a terrible poker face, despite her bad eyes, she notices. She swipes her hand, dismissing the irony of a Native American being a fan of a team with a name many indigenous people find offensive. "Politically correct hogwash!"

She's obviously quite comfortable expressing what's on her mind, as well as, apparently, given to suddenly changing course. "They thought I was a goner, you know?"

"Excuse me?"

"I'm talking about one of my times in the hospital, last year."

"Sounds scary."

"I was at peace, though. Ready to go. Wanting to go . . ."

She's drifted off to such an intimate place, I don't know what to do or say, other than remain, and appear, attentive. I try to summon up Rosalie's *Dos* and *Don'ts* for guidance, but they're all a-jumble.

"But then—I just wake up. I guess I'm just hard to get rid of."

"How fortunate I am that you're so stubborn!"

"Why do I get the sense we share this trait?"

"Maybe because I told you I'm half Polish?"

"Hah! To my one-quarter Mono!"

After ninety minutes, though her granddaughter Maymie's letter is never mentioned, she says, "I'm tired."

"Okay." I rise from the sofa. "I'll let you rest. I'll ring you in a few days."

"Do that. No guarantees, but . . ."

"Fair enough. But . . . would you like me to have a look at your letter?"

"Why not?" She nods toward a nearby TV tray.

My index finger touches a brown folder. "This it?"

Another nod.

"May I take it with me to work on it? Is this your only copy?"

"Sure. If you like. It is my only copy, but I trust you."

"Thank you. I'll keep it safe. Promise." I grab the folder and head toward the door but then turn around. "Oh, one question?"

"Fire away."

"Would you prefer that I call you Mrs. Burris or Mary Louise?"

"Why, haven't you been brought up properly!"

I smile.

"To answer your question, neither."

"Neither?"

"I'd actually prefer being called what I was called originally, by my tribe. I figure if it was good enough for my people, then it ought to be good enough for me."

"Okay. What were you called?"

"They called me Little One."

"Little One?"

She tells me it was the practice of the Mono not to name children until something "fit." Though eventually called Lena, until the age of seven her mother was called, simply, Little One. "As was I."

"The Little One it'll be, then."

"You can drop the definite article. 'Little One' will do just fine."

"Very well, then. Until next time, Little One." I step out into the hall.

"Hold on," she calls out.

I step back inside. "Yes?"

"What's good for the goose . . . How shall I refer to you? Mr. Lindner? Eric?"

"Whatever makes you feel more comfortable. But if you're asking me what I'm more comfortable with? . . ."

"That I am."

"Then it's Eric."

"Bye, Eric."

"Bye, Little One." I leave with the folder containing the letter to her six-year-old granddaughter. I also leave with some clothes she wants dry cleaned, which she wore to the funeral of her best friend, the mother of her daughter-in-law. My report includes the following excerpt:

> Sharp mind. Lots of spunk. Delightful! Patient says she needs more Xanax.

The next day, at home, I open the folder and remove its contents. In addition to some scribbled-on scraps of paper, there are nine hand-written pages. The letter begins:

> A letter to Mary Ann Burris, from her grandmother, Mary Louise Burris.
>
> Dear Maymie:
> That's the name given to you by your 1st cousin, Caroline Austin, when she couldn't say Mary Ann . . .

The cursive is smooth, self-assured. An absence of ink blobs suggest little stopping and starting. Thirteen self-corrections are small, such as a strike-through to change a verb tense, while three margin comments say "to be c/fied," "to be c/fied," and "Rewrite this page!!" Though generally neat, there is some evidence of fatigue: the upward drift appearing on page six gets worse toward the end, resulting in some sentences crossing lines.

Little One is clearly talented—all the more reason not to impose my own style on this treasured gift to her beloved granddaughter. I regard my role as organizational and administrative. I want to help her clarify her goals and objectives in order to get her points across. For starters, I digitize her work so she and I can follow it and edit it.

On my second visit, the first thing I do is stow her dry cleaning in the hallway closet. She calls over, "Tell me what I owe you."

"On the house," I say, as I make my way over to the sofa and sit beside her, beneath her papoose. "Want to talk about your letter a bit?"

"Let's."

I hand her a copy, printed in the eighteen-point font I use for my dad, whose macular degeneration is at least as bad as Mary Louise's. "Before turning to the printed stuff, how about you maybe just speak a few words, from the heart, about what it is you're trying to accomplish?"

"Excellent idea. Maymie reminds me a lot of my mother, and this is a good thing. My mother was born in eighteen ninety and lived to be ninety-nine. She was very clever and very beautiful. It was her beauty that scared people. She never wore any makeup—no lipstick, blush, nail polish. But she did 'dance like a dervish,' in a way that incited the young white men at the Saturday night square dances. Schizophrenically, the white parents tried to keep her hidden way—or marry her off."

"More of this sort of thing needs to be in your letter!"

"I know."

"Not to say you don't already have some great material. My favorite so far is this: 'My mother would tell of how she would climb a tree, staying all day, to avoid any white family that wanted to fix her up with one of their sons.' What a great image!"

She smiles. "So glad you like it. My mom was a real outdoors-woman. I imagine she could have held her own with—what was her name?—who went along with Lewis and Clark."

"Sacagawea." Though only sixteen and pregnant, Sacagawea was the only female on the expedition that played such a pivotal role in the development of this country.

"I bet she loved squirrel meat, too, like my mother. It was a real delicacy in nineteen twenty. Must have been Michelin three-star stuff in the early eighteen hundreds. I'll bet she also, like my mother, was adept at spearing the huge salmon that ran rampant in the rivers of central California when I was a child."

"But, obviously, your mom was lured out of her tree—the result being you."

"Yes, eventually. They got her to do lots of things. She started speaking English at the age of twelve, wearing makeup at thirty, and, the day before marrying, she became a Catholic."

Our collaboration is fun. I love her style, a distinctive, confidant mix of informal and formal, the latter evidenced by, for instance, her always referring to her granddaughter's letter as an "epistle," connoting its sanctity. We take turns talking, and listening, beneath the nineteenth-century Mono baby-hauling contraption on the wall above our heads, her ventilator mask more on than off. If I suggest some alternative diction or grammar, she'll nod, laugh, but also correct—if not reprimand—me. She'll shake her head, point at me, and snap, "No! You don't understand. Let me explain . . ."

Seeing as she's tired, as well as increasingly querulous, and I've got a few other things on my to-do list, I decide to shove off. Restowing the letter in its folder, I say, "I'll get cracking!"

It's during my third visit that Little One begins to open up a bit more about herself and not just her mother. The tales are tinged with darkness. "Life was hard as a quarter-breed. But I made something of myself. This is part of what I want to get across to Maymie. How to work through life's problems.

"The family who raised my mother and me gave us an awful lot, but they expected an awful lot, too. Emphasis on *awful*. 'Get on your knees!' I'll never forget the first time—of many—being yelled at. 'Get on your knees, and pray . . . for forgiveness and to be delivered from your heathen ignorance!'" Little One looks sad but also defiant.

"I doubt it was anything personal or racist . . ."

She stares at me—or glares, which I infer to mean, *How the hell would you know*??

Her arresting candor resumes on my fourth visit, with her response to my opening question, "So, how're things going for you today?"

"I've been in and out of the hospital nine times over the previous twelve months."

Clearly, she's uninterested in limiting the topic to today. "Gosh, that sounds rough."

"It has been. Now, pretty much, I'm a prisoner in this room here. Except for my TV. And this baby." She pats the oxygen tank. "And the Oxyfast ampules I squirt into the back of my throat when I feel like I can't breathe. And, of course, I've got my son, Jimmy . . ."

Jim's a high-tech services marketing guru. Apparently, though he's worked for some big companies and hit home runs, now he's on his own, as a consultant. He's also a recovering alcoholic. Sober for decades, he's a fixture at several local AA venues. "These days he thinks I'm the addict. Ha! He thinks I use oxycodone not so much because I can't breathe but because I like the high it produces. The escape it facilitates. Hooey."

The relationships the terminally ill have with their attending family members are often complex and inscrutable. The knot in this mother-son relationship is impossible to overlook.

Yet the love seems intact. I sense Jim's got a busy life. Plus, he's still reeling from the recent, sudden death of his mother-in-law. Yet still he visits his mom every Thursday, after a full shopping run. "Jimmy gets me everything I can possibly need and then some."

Despite her hints of aggravation and irritation, Little One is clearly very proud of her only child. "At Lora Beth's funeral, two women come up to me. I'd never laid eyes on them. One says, 'Mrs. Burris, I just wanted to tell you what a wonderful son you have!' 'Jim saved my life!' says the second. Until that moment, I had no idea Jimmy was so involved in AA . . . in helping . . . others. I just thought he sat around all day, fiddling with computers in his basement home office. Yet these ladies tell me that for many years, my Jimmy's been leading meetings twice a week. And that he's sponsored lots and lots of alcoholics. He's done and is doing so much good. Yet," she adds, mournfully, "I didn't know."

Khalil Gibran said, "Pain breaks the shell that encloses understanding." But what the great Lebanese mystic failed to note was that the emotional filling within the shell is seldom soft or sweet, like ripe Sidon figs. The more I get to know Little One and her son, the more I wonder what "filling" lay in store.


## APRIL 22

While working at home, on draft 2, a natural architecture begins to unfold around a set of picaresque experiences. Later, I drop by Little One's apartment, hand her my revision, and ask her to have a look. As she does, I wander around her apartment, pausing to admire her collection of gorgeous, valuable Native American basketry.

"Bingo!" she exclaims. "You've got it, exactly!" First, she wants to relate something about Maymie's provenance.

While you were delivered by a medical doctor, at a hospital, in a sterile room, imagine: my mother was delivered without the aid of any trained experts, by her grandmother, in the tepee they shared.

Second, Little One wants to alert Maymie to the bitter truth that life will be filled with myriad struggles and tragedies.

My father disappeared in 1919. In spite of extensive searches . . . his disappearance remains a mystery to this day. I remember struggling with how to make the *wh* sounds (such as in *where* and *who*). I was the only 'half-breed' in my class in elementary school (others were either full-blooded Native Americans or whites) . . . I recall having great difficulty with algebra.

Little One's third goal is to assemble a collection of tips in the hope of improving the chances that Maymie's joys will exceed her heartaches. Her first tip extols the virtue of friendship.

Your mother's lovely mother and I were "best friends" in the truest sense of the word. Our friendship was filled with respect and devotion. [She] used to bring me coffee every single day, help me run errands, and, most especially, provide companionship, as I did for her.

Another tip touches on love, marriage, and dancing.

Edward was a wonderful husband, in addition to which he was a wonderful dancer. *Important*. We danced a lot, even in the kitchen at 5:00 A.M. while preparing breakfast to the music of the radio.

Little One closes out the third section by stressing the importance of hard work.

Aunt Laura wasn't easy to work for . . . but a series of people saw me work, seemed to like my personality, and offered me jobs . . . While I never went to the sort of four-year college your parents attended . . . I worked my way up . . . in the War Department . . . to the Office of the Comptroller.

In her fourth and final section, Little One pours on the love.

Maymie, dear, you are a lovely child, blessed with loving parents, intelligent beyond your years, and ever so well behaved. Not only that, you are beautiful to look at. I have your picture everywhere. The whole family is so proud of you. You have never disappointed any of us.

I love you so much,

Your Nana

Her epistle seems on its way to becoming a beautiful bequest, far more meaningful and valuable than the mammon I'm familiar with in my circle of society.

But all is not rosy. I'm beginning to pick up that Jim's not thrilled with our progress, as if, having himself opened Pandora's box, he's now frantically trying to shut it, seal it, and bury it—deep. Why, I haven't a clue. Though he's the one who'd asked for a companion caregiver, and felt a letter to Maymie was a great idea, for his daughter as well as his mother, now, for some reason, he doesn't seem so keen on the fruits of my companionship.

Heeding Rosalie's *Do* to inform the entire caregiving team especially if and when something seems amiss, my April 22 report includes the following query and concern:

Especially confidential: is there some "issue" with her son that I should know about? Perhaps Lee might ring me?

## APRIL 24

Jim and I have yet to meet. But that doesn't stop me from forming an opinion, thereby breaching—yet again—this tip of Rosalie's: *Don't make assumptions.*

Jim's not at all shy about venting his spleen. When I ring him to discuss how and when to complete the epistle, given my hectic travel schedule, he unloads on his mom, calling her "an addict" for wanting so much pain medication and "spoiled" for having wasted her money yet now wanting to "live like a queen." During his diatribe, it occurs to me that never does he refer to my patient as *Little One*, *Mom*, *Mother*, or even *Mary Louise*, just *her* or *she*.

Later in the day, I arrive to find Little One preoccupied, perhaps regarding Jim. But she's more guarded (or more shy) than her son, not yet ready to entrust me with her most precious, sensitive—vulnerable—thoughts. She says she doesn't feel like working on the epistle, so Maymie's gift stalls. But she utters a few remarks, seemingly against her will. "I don't know what Jimmy does all day, but he makes it seem like a big production, his coming by to bring me some money. He's the one who slashed my allowance, who took away my cell phone."

I detect more fatigue than rancor. Little One has clearly begun to slip, somatically and mentally. Though mostly listless, confiding that she's "anxious," at times she gets agitated, saying she's "terror stricken." Today's report includes the following excerpt:

> Poor thing seems so alone. Perceives° herself to be abandoned by the death of her best friend, indifference°° of son.
>
> ° my opinion °° not saying he is in fact indifferent

Once I'm home, Lee Lund rings me. The Haymarket Hospice social worker sheds some additional light on the situation: "Jim's really angry—at something."

I wonder if his ire is directed at me—say, that by bringing Little One coconut patties from a Florida airport or apple turnovers from the local grocery store I'm contributing to her being spoiled and living like a queen. My suspicion seems supported by the fact that though I've called him a few times (getting through once, earlier this same day) he's never called me.

"No," Lee insists, "I thought that, too, that he was mad at me. But it's not you, me, or us. There's something else going on, and we happen to have walked right into the middle of it."

## APRIL 29

I bring along draft 3, setting her copy on the TV tray table. She ignores it. Despite considerable progress, the epistle remains in flux. We've a long way to go, and, I fear, not much time.

Patient in tough shape. Really laboring re: breathing.

Very anxious.


## MAY 6

Little One rallies, at least temperamentally. However, her epistle is still plagued by meandering and patches of indecipherability. Whereas a week earlier I'd left her with five neat pages (in my twelve-point font), she hands me back, in addition to my typed pages—copiously marked up—two brand new handwritten pages along with a small bundle of scribblings jotted on Post-Its, random scraps of paper, etc.

Her work almost seems that of several different people, but I realize it's probably just the effects of her oxycodone, creeping Alzheimer's, and the like. She mixes blue and black ink. Some writing is perfectly legible, other passages are inscrutable thickets, and still others in between, as evidenced by the following, jotted at the top of page three:

Add to Mother's—fun—make it funny.

"I've certainly got my hands full!" I say as I'm gathering my things, preparing to leave her apartment. As I pass by the kitchen, where her meds and an instruction sheet are located, I say, in passing, "You okay for meds?"

Companion caregivers have no business meddling in meds. It is strictly forbidden, a cardinal *Don't* that Rosalie hammered away at during orientation. I've never asked such a question of any other patient.

But Little One is unlike any other patient in so many ways, including her honestly telling me that she felt terror stricken when all my other patients, as a general rule, have tried to deny or hide their fears. "I'm not sure," she says. "Could you check, please?"

So I check. "Looks like you've got one ampule prepared."

Though it's been off for the duration of my visit, now she frantically gropes for her oxygen mask. Just before strapping it on, she says, her tone steeped in anxiety, "Just one?"

I've seen enough patients panic attacking to know that if it gets rolling it's like a runaway train. The key is not letting the train start to roll. But it's too late. Little One's Panic Train has already left the station. Instructions in the kitchen (though on a blank white sheet, I presume they were typed by a Haymarket Hospice professional) say she can take one ampule hourly, yet all she's got on hand is one dose to last her twenty hours, including through the night.

A key Haymarket Hospice service metric is "total pain control within seventy-two hours." Well, an RN I'm not. An MD I am not. But something's been poorly controlled. Moreover, I know that emotional, psychic fear can be as acutely painful as any physical, somatic trauma. Indeed, pain's multidimensional nature is the philosophical foundation of hospice care.

Perhaps I should ring Maureen Samet, RN, or Rosalie Palermo and discuss the situation. After all, I signed a legal document acknowledging the strictly limited, nonmedical nature of my role (as an unskilled companion)—such an acknowledgment precisely designed to prevent me from even considering what I'm now debating.

My mind's lost in a maze of fuzzy ambivalence, hedged by a few clear, narrow paths. The federal HIPAA laws are clear, as is the volunteer agreement I signed, but so are the kitchen instructions. What's involved here is not the illicit use of a controlled substance but the lack of a licit dosage. Also, while there's a big *Do Not Resuscitate* sign on the front door of her apartment, this isn't on point, for I'm not thinking about resuscitating her.

Could she fill the ampules herself? I know she's done so in the past. But these days, with her hands so trembly, her eyesight so compromised? If her nurse typically fills them, or Jim, why isn't there an adequate supply on hand?

An even worse thought creeps into the equation: convinced his mom's an addict, is Jim unilaterally suppressing her palliative relief? Is what's going on here—perhaps—suggestive of abuse, implicating the vital *Do* of letting Rosalie know?

On the other hand, Jim's known Little One for forty-nine years, and his being clean and sober for the past eighteen makes it crystal clear to him that his mom should not be taking—or be given—this powerful drug. Yet here I come along, having spent maybe twenty hours with his mom—giving serious thought to overruling his vastly superior experience as well as one of Haymarket Hospice's cardinal *Don'ts*.

Meanwhile, Little One begins panting, hyperventilation's first gear. Her eyes bulge as she strains to suck more air than the thin plastic tubing can transport.

Could she be faking it? Is she "playing" me? This prompts a final consideration: trust. To me, *faith* doesn't mean blindly adhering to some dogma but knowing someone's got your back, having total confidence in more than something—someone. If Little One can't trust me, what am I doing in her apartment? Why am I volunteering? She's entrusted me with, arguably, the most important thing in her life: her epistle. Isn't it right that I extend some quid pro quo?

Right or wrong, I prepare five ampules, just 25 percent of the permissible dosage. I'm very careful in measuring out the powerful oxycodone, using an eyedropper.

Still . . . the moment I leave . . . could Little One hobble up and over, guzzle all five at once, and die? Possibly. Have I taken the law into my own hands? The jury's out on that one.

## MAY 7

My cell phone rings a little before noon. I don't recognize the number. Atypically, but as I did when Jay rang me in Poland, to inform me about Dolly, I decide to answer. "Hello?"

"I'm trying to get ahold of Eric Lindner?" The woman sounds nice, but tentative, like she'd drawn the short end of the stick.

"That's me."

"Oh. This is Mara Forsten, from Haymarket Hospice."

"Hi, Mara." Uh-oh. At first her name doesn't ring a bell, but then I recall having received an e-mail recently introducing her as a new assistant volunteer coordinator. But why's Rosalie—the head coordinator—not calling me? Have I gotten her in trouble?? No question I felt repercussions were possible. Okay, probable. But I didn't expect them to materialize so fast.

"I'm calling regarding one of your patients, Mary Louise Burris."

"Little One."

"Huh?"

"That's the name she prefers. Not Mary Louise."

"Uh . . . okay, I guess."

My ploy is deliberate, using Mary Louise's Native name to obfuscate. Maybe it'll cause Mara to question her facts, on which her impending reprimand (or so I presume) is based. "What about Little—?"

Suddenly my sophistry is rent by a thunderclap thought: How do I know this is just a reprimand? My question explodes into shrapnel. Is Little One dead?? Have I killed her?? Would Jim come after me? How about Haymarket Hospice? How about Virginia's Department of Social Services? Do I need a defense attorney? Should I call Kathy Roach? Warren Nowlin? Would the commonwealth prosecutor want to make an example of me? Would my umbrella policy cover me, or would my carrier say my having acted "with intent" precludes coverage and prevail in a lawsuit lasting years and costing me an arm and a leg—contractually and financially impaling me like a jiggling, idiotic, non-practicing attorney . . . headed straight toward . . . along Good Intentions Boulevard—hell. I'd better call Kathy and Warren and get them on a conference call! What will Ellen say? What will my folks think? Holy shi—!

"You really shouldn't be giving her any meds. We don't want you to get into a lot of legal trouble, now do we?"

"So . . ." I'm not in "a lot" already? "Then . . . she's . . . okay?"

"Your patient? Why yes, she's fine. So far as I know. Thanks for all you do. Bye now."

A few hours later, I buzz Little One from the entrance to her apartment complex. "Hel . . . loooo?" she answers, over the intercom. There's a distinctively impish tone to her voice.

It's so great to hear your voice! "It's Eric. Can I pop up for a minute?" I fib as to why: "While at the store, I saw the baker wheel out some fresh apple turnovers, your favorite." The truth is I want to set my eyes on her. Also, if she's experienced any blowback occasioned by my filling of the ampules, I'd like to try and clean up the mess I've made.

"I'll buzz you in. I've got a surprise for you too!"

Once upstairs, I knock on the door to her unit. As always, it's ajar.

"Come on in!" She sounds happy, revved up.

I enter. She's in her chair, beneath her papoose. Jim Burris is pacing in front of the TV.

I freeze, arms akimbo, holding two plastic shopping bags. I'm terrible with names and dates, and everything like that. It's my wife who must always remind me to send my mom a birthday card, for example. I've forgotten that this is Thursday, Jim's day to visit. Under ordinary circumstances, it's much better for me to spread out the coverage, as well as to allow Little One some time alone with her own flesh and blood. That these are extraordinary circumstances—namely, that I've just defied the wishes of this ex-junkie and alcoholic by preparing five doses for his mother, "the addict"—makes our first meeting all the more charged.

This is my first time laying eyes on him. He appears about my age (early fifties) and height (6'2"), but he's thinner, wiry. He's in blue jeans and sneakers. He looks more focused and coiled than pissed—like a cobra about to strike. He avoids looking at me as he rearranges the TV tray beside his mom, shuffling the remote, her hairbrush, and the folder containing her epistle.

There's mutual discord. To me, he's the son who's ignored his terrified, terminally ill mom's pleas for palliative relief as well as, most likely, the one behind Mara's reprimand. To him, I'm a pusher, supplying his mom with drugs she shouldn't have. After battling his own addictions for decades, while he's out helping other people battle theirs, in slips Trojan Horse me, exacerbating his already-strained relationship with his mom. On top of everything else, now I'm intruding on his regular day to visit. I'm guessing that, at this moment, he rues ever having called Haymarket Hospice, speaking with Rosalie, and asking for a volunteer.

Neither of us makes a move toward the other. Nor do we appear the least bit interested in smiling or shaking hands. Clearly we're both struggling to be civil and play nice.

Clearly Little One wishes we'd not. She half-giggles, half-rasps, 100 percent the happy provocateur.

Though his pacing has slowed somewhat, Jim's still avoiding my eyes when he says, "We appreciate all that you're doing for Mary Louise."

"Sorry about filling her meds," I say, reciprocating if not an entire olive branch at least a sprig. "Believe me, I got Mara's message loud and clear!"

Our cordiality causes Little One to pout. "Hogwash! I'm glad you filled them!"

Jim stops pacing and snaps his neck at his mother. His eyes widen and flash. But knowing he's outnumbered two to one, he bristles impotently while rearranging the TV tray table, for the umpteenth time. "You did a good job," he mutters. "I will say that. Very precise."

This is my cue to leave. "I don't want to horn in on your day with your son, Little One," passively aggressively not even referring to Jim by name and calling her Little One, when he's just referred to her as Mary Louise. "Just that, as I said I would, when I'm at the grocery store, if I see fresh apple turnovers, the type I know you like, I'll grab them. I saw some today, so I'll just leave them here in the kitchen. Nice meeting you, Jim," I lie. *Jerk.*

"Nice meeting you, Eric," he lies back. *Asshole.*

## MAY 8

There's a new Notice! tacked up in the kitchen. It's a curt reminder "to all caregivers" that only Little One's nurse or doctor is permitted to refill her ampules. Signed by an MD, it's on Haymarket Hospice letterhead. Having written my share of ex post facto cover-your-ass missives, here's my take on what the notice really means:

Dear Mr. Burris and the law firm we suspect you have already retained,

Rest assured: the health and safety of every patient is Haymarket Hospice's number one priority. We have taken great pains to ensure that all of our volunteers are thoroughly trained and constantly reminded what their role is—and is not. However, if some jackass volunteer ignores the aforementioned and entirely adequate training, in contravention of our explicit rules and regulations, while we are terribly sorry, naturally, we cannot be held accountable.

Look to the jackass for relief.

Have a nice day,

The Haymarket Hospice Legal Department & the law firm of Caggiula & Loeber, Where Every Client Is a Deep Pocket®

While reading the notice, I call over to Little One, "Guess I'm in the dog house, huh?"

"I guess you are! You and me both."

"Don't you find, sometimes, it's nice being sent outside, into the fresh air?"

"You said it! They're awfully cheap with their medicine, you ask me. I didn't touch what you left me. But it sure put my mind at ease. Thank you again."

"Tell me, how much does Jim hate me?"

She bats away the question. "He'll get over it."

Meanwhile, I'm trying to be a good son myself as well as be there for my own son and daughter. Or am I? When I force myself to confront Jung's "shadow," to drill down into that brackish well of honesty I'd prefer were kept capped, I'm not so sure how much I'm trying, really. My priorities seem askew. Jim Burris seems to wish that I'd never entered his life, yet I've foisted myself upon him, whereas my family needs me, and I'm so often AWOL.

I'm struggling to help my parents make the sort of lifestyle changes that, though they may seem simple and logical, are in fact rarely easy (e.g., giving up the car). Also, I want to do my share of shuttling them to doctor appointments in D.C. and Baltimore. And I need to be there for them when an ambulance is their shuttle to the ER, which is happening much more frequently.

I'm also struggling to help my son find his way in the world, as a twenty-one-year-old. Problem is, I'm hardly the best guide for Matt, given my track record at his age. In certain ways, he's already very much a man— big and burly, he towers over me in our Christmas card photo, and I'm 6'2", 185 pounds. What's more, he's been a committed community service volunteer far longer than I—as a first responder, rushing into burning buildings, and pulling tire-screeching U-turns when he happens upon gory traffic accidents. In one year alone he made some sixty "runs" while a full-time high school student, while studying, on his own, on the side, to earn his Firefighter I certificate. One such run led to a commendation letter from his fire chief for bravery above and beyond. Matt's also a genuinely humble kid: Ellen and I were unaware of his heroics until his chief's letter arrived in the mail. My wife and I are very proud of him.

However, since high school Matt's been struggling with what he wants to do, where he wants to do it, with whom. He needs more guidance from me. Problem is, I'm no Sacagawea.

I tell Little One about Matt. "He's looking for a new type of college program, one more focused on battling wildfires, outdoors, as opposed to structure fires, in urban settings. We've stumbled across this place in California's Central Valley. Reedley College has this outstanding forestry and wildlife management program. Know where it is?"

"I know exactly where it is," she says. "It's just down the road from where I was born!"

"No kidding??"

"No, I am not kidding. And my recommendation to you is this: Go! It's God's country. You'll not see anything like it, anywhere."

So, after my thirteenth visit, it's westward ho on a thirteen-day cross-country trip with my son, leaving Little One all alone to cope with hers.

While traveling with Matt, however, it's a different ninety-four-year-old who helps me the most: Dolly, whom I've been seeing in parallel with Little One. Dolly's been teaching me how to communicate better. By my trekking with him, Matt sees he's a top priority—far more effectively than all my words to this effect, in stacks of letters and memos, and years of heart-to-heart talks.

## JUNE 8

Once back from California, as I'm about to head over to her apartment one afternoon, Little One calls in advance. "I'm at Fauquier Hospital." She sounds fine, but she can't be.

"What?? Why? How are you?"

"Well, they're running tests on me now. The doctor says I've still got all my wits about me. But I didn't need him to tell me that. My leg's sure a mess, though."

She goes on to explain how, a few days earlier, she'd tried to clip a toe nail. Poor, half-blind thing, she'd mangled the job. An infection set in. Now, not just her foot but her entire left leg is a mess. "It's quite a sight," she says. "It's in Technicolor."

When I arrive at the hospital, I detour into the gift shop. The perfect gift is soon staring me in the face: a stuffed baby black bear. It's as if a cub had stowed away on my flight from the Fresno Yosemite International Airport.

She's asleep when I arrive at her room. Her leg looks terrible. Horribly swollen, it's a discolored patchwork of orange, brown, purple, and black. Hooked up to oxygen, a mask over her mouth and nose, her breathing is labored, phlegmy.

A nurse enters. "You family?"

I shake my head. "Haymarket Hospice. Name's Eric."

She studies me for a moment, perhaps looking for my ID tag, which I never wear. The bear seems to allay any lingering doubts. "How cute." She pulls up close to Little One, gently tufts her pillow, and strokes her hair. "Poor dear. In and out of consciousness. When awake, she's hallucinating half the time. But this morning, she did ask for her hair to be done. We'll see if she remembers." After a final glance at Little One's leg and vitals, the nurse departs.

I take a seat in the cramped room's only chair, and, as my eyes wander, Little One clears her throat and rustles her sheets. I stand, walk over to her, and rest a hand on her shoulder.

As her glasses are off, she's totally blind. The mask muffles her words. "Who's that?"

"Eric."

"Who?"

"Here." I hand her glasses to her. It takes her a while to get them on, after which she gives me the up-down. I'm not sure she recognizes me. Maybe she's back at Strategic Air Command, denying some low-level officer access to the top brass.

"You were right. That part of California . . . I couldn't believe how gorgeous it is."

She's studying me intently, trying to get her bearings. Her brown eyes are filmy, riven by tiny red veins.

I hand her the bear. "A little something from back home."

Comprehension dawns. She chokes up as her mask flops to her collarbone. "Oh! . . ."

"When I saw this . . . made in a Chinese sweatshop, modeled after a California bear, sold in a Virginia hospital. How's that for destiny?"

She hugs her new companion and cries. Tears slip under her glasses, pooling in the upturned oxygen mask, overflowing, dribbling onto the bear's backside. As she wicks them away, tenderly, protectively, like a mother wanting to prevent a cold, my stomach does a bittersweet back flip.

I hold up the folder, containing draft 4. "On the flight home, I read over the latest additions to your epistle. As usual, I really like what you've done!"

She ignores me, or doesn't hear me. She's too busy snuggling her bear. She extends her arms as if appraising a newborn baby, as she undoubtedly appraised Jim. "What shall I call you?" A finger goes to her lips. "Hmmm. I know! I shall call you Monahu."

"'Hello' in your native tongue, right?"

Now, for the first time during this visit, our eyes really connect. She seems totally with it. "That's right, Eric. You've been a good student."

I fake a frown. "I can't leave you alone for two weeks without your going and getting yourself in trouble??"

"What can I say? I'm a natural-born troublemaker."

"I can't thank you enough for encouraging me to take Matt to the land of the Mono."

"Didn't I tell you you'd fall in love with my ancestral homeland?"

"Yes, you did. Still, I thought you might have been exaggerating a bit."

"I may be a troublemaker, but I'm not an exaggerator."

I nod toward the TV. CNN's *Headline Sports* is muted. "How're the Nats doing?"

"Great." Her tone is jaunty. "They're several games above five hundred. Which is a whole heck of a lot better than I'm doing, that's for sure."

When *Headline News* resumes, I nod at Obama. Before a podium, his back is to a sea of gray-clad Army cadets.

"I saw him today." She lifts the mask to her face to take a pull of oxygen.

"I see he was up at West Point delivering a commencement speech."

Suddenly agitated, she yanks off her mask. "You don't understand! I was there."

"You were . . ." Uh-oh.

"After I did the laundry, cleaned the kitchen, and ran some errands. Just now sat down—okay, lay down—for the first time today, just before you got here. And . . . they're talking to me."

"Who's talking to you?"

She wags a finger in the direction of the TV, at the talking head. "Them. On TV. They're asking me questions. Of course they can't hear my answers."

"'Course not."

Then her fog lifts. "So . . . you like my letter, do you?"

"Absolutely! I love it!"

"I'm glad. Really glad." She returns the mask to her face, and closes her eyes.

I visit her four times over the next fourteen days, staying, on average, about an hour. Reminiscent of my final visits with Bob, I'm not sure if she's asleep, but her eyes are closed. She looks the same each time, as does her epistle . . . apparently untouched since my return from California . . .

The epistle is, maybe, two-thirds complete. There's much Little One still wants to say, floating around inside her head, a head getting less coherent by the hour. At this rate, I seriously doubt it'll be finished in time, which means I'll have failed in my primary mission.

She never makes it back to her apartment. Instead, she's shipped straight to a nursing home. I shouldn't visit her. Nursing homes are off limits to me. I'm still not fully recovered from the bad infection that, most likely, I either contracted or exacerbated in the course of visiting another ninety-four-year-old female patient at a different nursing home.

## JUNE 22

I can't abandon Little One. I don't tell my wife, but . . . to hell with my eye.

I arrive to a sad, antiseptic place, of squeaky wheelchairs and blank stares. I've brought flowers: a big, colorful bouquet. Once in her room, after sliding the countertop TV to one side, I tuck the arrangement into the corner so it faces her.

She's groggy. Her oxygen mask is off: a good sign, unexpected. I wonder, could Little One be the one, finally, who rallies? After all, one out of every six hospice patients is a "live discharge," and, though I've had a dozen patients, I've yet to see one return to the mainstream of life. I'm due. Plus, like Dolly, Little One is deceptively tough and resilient. "Who's there?"

"It's Eric." I squeeze her hand.

"Who? Why am I here? I don't want to be here!"

"I'm sorry. Can I do something for you?"

"Make sure it's a best-seller."

"Excuse me?" At the time, though my wife and a few close friends have been urging me to write about my hospice experiences, Little One knows nothing about such thinking. Yet, somehow, she does know . . .

"Your book, silly. About me and Monahu. Once you finish my epistle, then, you must finish your gospel. Send an autographed copy to Monahu and to Jim."

"Uh . . . Okay."

For the remainder of my visit, she flits and floats amongst lucidity, confusion, and hallucination. "Monahu's hungry. He misses home. I

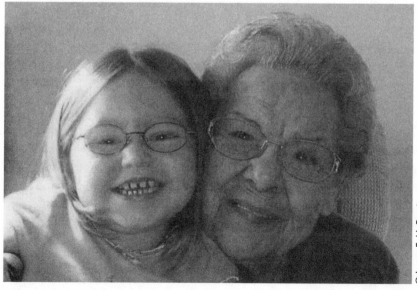

© James E. H. Burris

hate the Yankees! I need my nails done. My foot hurts! Why hasn't Obama returned my call? Get my latest edits from Jimmy. I like the changes you made. Jimmy read them to me. Wish Matt good luck."

Her eyes lock onto mine as she says, "You run along now."

## JUNE 25

Just as I'm leaving home, sneaking out the laundry room door, on another covert nursing home visit, Rosalie calls. I whisper, "Yes?"

"She's gone."

I lean against the doorframe. "Poor thing. I'm really going to miss her. But thanks for letting me know. This must be one of the hardest parts of your job, huh?"

"It is. And, I'm afraid, I've got something else I need to tell you. I'm leaving Haymarket Hospice. It's time."

Time? . . . Time for what? Her statement is pregnant with potential meaning, but as our relationship hasn't quite yet crossed that professional-personal border, I decide it would be inappropriate to probe. But the news saddens me and worries me. Has her cancer returned?

"I'm being replaced by Mara Forsten. You'll like her. I know you two have talked."

"Yes, we did. But, Rosalie! I hope we'll stay in touch?"

"I hope so."

## JUNE 26

The next day I get a call from Jim Burris. "I just wanted to make sure you'd heard. Mary Louise passed. She made me promise to tell you, especially." He laughs. It's a short burst, more expulsion of air than expression of levity.

"Yes, Jim, thanks. Haymarket Hospice informed me. I'm so sorry. Will there be a service of some sort? If so, I'd like to attend and pay my respects."

"Nope. No service. Apart from us, and you, Mary Louise really didn't have anyone. But . . . she was adamant that I make sure to get her final notes to you so she—you, I suppose—can finish her letter to my daughter.

"Is . . ." Jim continues, sounding puzzled, embarrassed, "gosh . . . is it fair of me to even ask that you see this through? I mean . . . it would mean so much to my daughter . . . and to me."

"'Course it's fair. And not just fair. Right. But it's *her* letter, Jim. One hundred percent."

"Yeah. I read your notes to her. I like your approach."

That evening, Jim e-mails me the short obituary, which concludes,

> If there is a heaven, she's probably already enjoying a Manhattan (and a smoke) with her big guy.

A few weeks later, as arranged, on my way into D.C. I pop by Jim's house and collect a packet of materials from his wife. This is the first time Susan and I have ever spoken to one another, let alone met. She kindly invites me in for coffee.

"I'd love to, but I got lost finding this place. Not on account of your directions, trust me! But I'm late for a meeting downtown. Can I get a rain check? Once I'm finished and send you the final version of Little One's—"

She scrunches up her nose, only knowing of her mother-in-law as Mary Louise.

"—uh . . . Mary Louise's letter, maybe we can get together for coffee or lunch?"

"That'd be great."

"And I'm so sorry for your other loss, too. Your mother. You've taken some real hits as of late."

Her eyes fall to the curb. "Yeah. Like . . . yeah. It's been rough."

A few days later, I open the envelope Susan gave me. Little One's final scribblings are a hodgepodge. While at times her longhand retains its elegant flow and is easy to follow, there's also a fair bit of chicken scratch.

Fortunately, I'm able to decipher some final revisions, including in the opening sentence of the first of two new handwritten pages, "Mother had a wonderful sense of curiosity. She was interested in everything." Thus begins a terrific new anecdote, illustrating Little One's counsel of curiosity, via an adventurous spirit, pursuant to a journey along Route 66—with her mother, in a jalopy, back in the '40s, even though neither had a license or had ever ventured out of the State of California. "Mother just surmised that I would handle all the details. Correct, as usual." The deerskin-clad Mono girls were in stitches all the way, despite sweating all the way, until fashioning a makeshift air conditioner from a hunk of dry ice they'd finagled from a Mormon missionary gas station owner in Utah, sealing the deal by agreeing to read *The Book of Mormon*, which they do, in rapt amusement, learning how Jesus returned to Latin America and appeared before a new set of apostles, some Native American cousins of theirs, down in Peru or thereabouts. "We had a ball."

Paper-clipped to the first sheet are some scribbled-on scraps of Navajo code-talk for all I know and a second handwritten page, nearly identical to the first but for a word here and there. For instance, while the second repeats "Mother had a wonderful sense of curiosity," it follows with a sentence that is scribbled over and stricken through numerous times, but, still, I can make out as saying either "Sometimes she drove me crazy" or "Sometimes she made me cry." My guess is Little One meant to say she laughed so hard she cried, but I can't be sure. But as the neater first page seems to govern, neither the "cry" nor "crazy" sentence makes it into the final version of the epistle, which comes in at five and a half pages.

## OCTOBER 3, 2012

Twenty-seven months after Little One's death Jim and I are having our second lunch together at our favorite Lebanese restaurant. We're sharing a laugh over how we misjudged each other, how our families were thrown together, to help each other. "Jim, I can't thank you enough."

Hearing Little One recount Jim's brave battle with alcoholism led me to confront my own overindulgence. Since not drinking for more than two and a half years, I'm more alert and healthier overall. (More popular, too, being the perennial designated driver.)

My son's transformed, too. Succumbing to the magical land of the Mono, embracing the Native American respect for the sanctity of Nature, his unique purpose in life snaps into focus, gelling around forestry, firefighting, wildlife management, and conservation. He falls in love with—and, aces—material far afield from (and arguably far more worthwhile than) the sort of stuff I took in B-school and law school, course titles like dendrology, where he learns why fires are a natural part of Nature and thus shouldn't be fought—say for instance because a certain pinecone will only bloom and blossom at high temperatures—and wilderness survival, where he learns from an ex-Navy SEAL that, for the most part, eating bugs with eight or more legs is, if not quite kosher, at least nutritious and palatable, but that the six-legged suckers'll give you a nasty case of the trots, at the very least. Matt also schools me on the difference between parks—"It's okay to hunt, and drive snowmobiles"—and forests—"Most stuff is off-limits." When we're driving together through the Sierra Nevada, Smoky, and Blue Ridge mountains, rather than rattling off the sort of pedantic legalisms my student cohort so loves to spout, Matt shares with me the Latin names of myriad redwoods, poplars, and willow-oaks. He lands a coveted apprenticeship with the National Park Service's last Back-Country Ranger, learns to track the old-school way (with a Greek compass, not a Garmin gadget), and tears around a track with a heavy backpack fast enough to get his Red Card, enabling him to fight fires from northern Maine to southern Kauai, in every U.S. forest and park.

As for Little One's son, reading her last words opens a door to closure, but, still, Jim's not there yet. "Mary Louise wasn't my birth mother."

"No kidding? So she was . . . your adoptive mother."

He shrugs while mopping up the last of the humus with a wedge of still-warm pita.

"When'd you find out?"

"I really began suspecting it just about the time you began volunteering."

"So that's what was going on! You seemed angry, or at least preoccupied with something that upset you, deeply, but I couldn't understand . . . Were you mad at your—uh, Mary Louise?"

"Yes. I was mad. Not so much now. But I'm still not totally over it. You've got to understand, everything I'd been told, everything about my background, was built on a lie. My daughter and I had a right to know the truth."

"That must have been rough. How'd you find out?"

"It wasn't easy. I got the public records, but California is one of forty-some states that still don't allow the adopted child to learn the actual identity of their birth parents. So I had to play detective."

"Know who your birth mom was, now?"

"My supposed aunt. My mom's sister. She was a wild child."

"You certain? I mean . . . I'd guess the names are redacted . . . ?"

"You'd guess right. But I knew enough about the general background: where Mary Louise was living, the age of her sister—my real mom— that sort of thing."

"She's mentioned in the letter."

"I know."

"Hidden in plain sight, maybe? And . . . pardon me if it sounds like I'm trying to defend Little One, but isn't it possible she made a solemn promise to her sister not to tell? And so she was truly on the horns of an ethical dilemma. I'd imagine it was hard on her. Tore her up inside."

"I've thought about that. Yes it's possible . . . maybe even likely. But still, I feel that, once my birth mom died, as she did a long time ago, Mary Louise had an overriding obligation to tell me the truth about my background. That she didn't, well . . ." His eyes wander. "Fortunately, I found this Internet e-mail support group called Late Discovery Adoptees. They've been great."

"I am really sorry about all this."

"Not your fault. I'll tell you what I can't understand. She took all this time to write a letter to my daughter—and it's a wonderful letter, too, don't get me wrong. Yet she doesn't take thirty seconds to tell me something that's at least as worthy of expression. It just caused, or at least contributed to, so much unhealthiness. We're only as sick as our secrets."

After our lunch, consistent with how I've tried to involve and respect the perceptions, desires, and dignity of all of my patients and their loved ones (which has at times proven to be quite a challenge, given the existence of so many different—valid—viewpoints), I send Jim the final draft of the chapter on Little One, soliciting his input. He responds immediately.

Eric—

First I want to say how wonderful the book has turned out. It's both literate and heartfelt and I'm grateful my mom and my family and I are in it. I thank you and I find it beautiful just as it is. It really works!

I laughed. I cried.

As to the former, your "Lawyer Letter" is brilliant! (I told you I really never gave a shit you did that for her . . . Filled those ampules . . . If anything I'm grateful—it saved me a trip!!!)

Now to the latter . . . It's with real reluctance that I tell you I am struggling with a couple parts of it . . . I'm going to put it all out here . . .

My difficulties with Mary Louise had been built over a lifetime of her making it painfully obvious to me that I fell short in absolutely everything I ever accomplished and more importantly, everything I ever did on her behalf.

While I'd had an inkling my whole life and it grew to a suspicion toward the end of hers, I didn't learn the truth of my adoption until almost a full year after Mary Louise's—okay, Little One . . . I've no desire to fight you on that, or her . . . But, Eric, don't you see the irony even in this . . . the further proof of my estrangement—initiated by *her*? She tells you—a stranger—about this desire of hers to be called by her Native American name . . . but the first *I* ever hear of it—is from you, after she dies!

I can tell you honestly, as a recovering, twenty-year medal man who only got to twenty by being honest: upon learning of my heritage . . . by far my main regret and concern was for my beloved Maymie . . . not knowing her true genetics and of course Little One's Big Lie. I've done a lot of work on forgiveness since . . . I am almost 100% of the way there.

But I digress . . .

The anger you may have *perceived* when you first met me was not anger—honestly . . . but rather just the manifestation of my being burnt out—to a crisp—in trying, and failing to satisfy . . . Little One.

Let me tell you something, Eric: Little One was big-time needy!—for attention, more visits with Maymie, time, always money, and of course love. There was never enough of anything for Little One. God knows we all tried. I can assure you Eric, when you saw me, you saw an exhausted and defeated man, on the *de*fensive . . . I'd never touched a loved one in anger, never acted out in any way violently or been verbally abusive to anyone in my family—EVER!

Little One was also a big-time spendthrift, whose eyes were way way WAY bigger than her little bank account. I did a financial intervention in 2005. It was Ripley's Believe It or Not! She'd run up more than $40,000 in credit card debt and acquired . . . we could never figure it out!!—100 pairs of shoes from QVC—check. But what else? Her family never saw it. I used the money from my birth mother's estate to pay off the cards. I took her cards away, and Little One never forgave me. I used what little money remained to move her from Maryland to Virginia so she could be closer to Susan's family and to us.

Then I spend months rehabbing her Maryland condo and put it on the market—just as the mortgage crisis hit. I carry the expenses, finally get it rented—at a loss—while I'm trying to start a company and take care of Susan and Maymie. Hell, M.L. never once said, "Thank you—fill in the blank." Was she conflicted about my status? Did she resent ever having assumed such a burden—i.e., me. Don't ask me! That's why the quacks get the big bucks!

And, as to her letter to Maymie? Let me tell you about another letter she wrote . . .

So I move her into The Oaks, just about throwing out my back in the process. Though a lovely place, full of nice people, upon my first return visit—saying not a word, M.L. slaps me with two typewritten pages of complaints. I shit you not. Once again: no thanking, just bitching.

Now, to her medical condition . . . We pre-interviewed doctors, told them of her disorders—not the least of which, factious disorder (akin to Munchausen's Syndrome), resulted in her actually researching disorders, manifesting physical symptoms, seeking medical attention, and collecting drugs. Let me rewind the tape a bit: while cleaning up her Maryland condo, I discover two black plastic lawn and leaf bags full of (no exaggeration!!) unused prescription drugs, from dozens of doctors. Maybe that was the source of those credit card balances?

Now, I ask you to reflect for a moment on the pathology of the above, as I've done for many years . . . How cagey she had to be to hornswoggle so many doctors . . . How she acquired so much stuff, but used so little of it . . . like it was—as I do think it was—just a game to her . . .

As she declined, the game grew uglier. She became more strident and brutal in her expressions of dissatisfaction, disappointment, and entitlement. I could handle it far better than Susan but, maybe, I didn't handle it so well. When Mary—Little—whatever!! started leveling her nastiness at Susan—who really burned out trying to off-load me and placate M.L.— your Little One crossed a big line with me. I had to step in and step it up. I resented having to do the job but did it with as much tolerance, love, and understanding as I could muster. I admit: I was worn down. Angry about my wife being hurt. That's what you saw . . . It was fresh, raw . . .

Eric, I really don't want this MOST IMPORTANT POINT to get lost in all my caterwauling: I really did love her, and still do.

TO REPEAT: I take NO issue whatsoever with your account of your time with . . . Little One. To me it's not about "this or that being true"— we're both right, both being truthful. Life's facts often look very different . . . the way the moon does . . . at different times . . . from different angles.

I know I've said it before, already, in person and in letters and e-mails, but: I'm truly happy and thankful . . . that you were able to bring some happiness to her near the end of her life. Everyone deserves happiness then. Little One was damaged, that's all. Like us all. Thank you.

Talk to you soon,

Jim

I respond immediately, via e-mail. Jim and I swap e-mails, talk over the phone. He closes things out, ever graciously, with the following e-mail:

Hi Eric—

No worries or heartburn at all on any of this! Your book is about **your** impressions and **your** experience . . . Just like M.L.'s letter was for her . . . It's your memoir, not a history—and I like it a lot.

Get in touch any time.

Peace & strength.

Jim

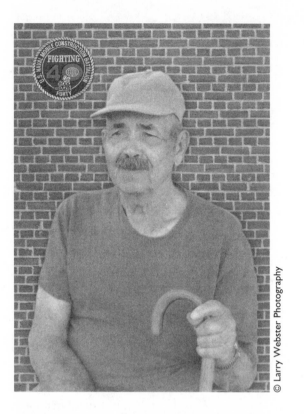

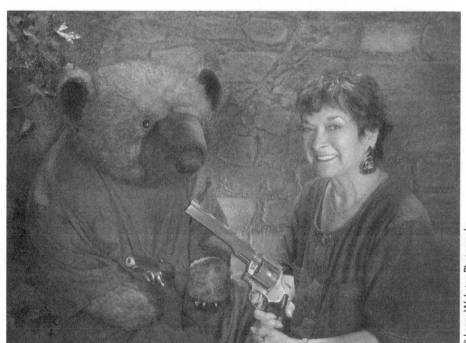

# HAVE GUNS, WILL TRAVEL

**W**ith booze subtracted from my life, I'm sleeping longer and, while awake, seemingly accomplishing twice as much. As forty-five years of accumulated toxins decompose, seep out, and evaporate, I'm resolving knotty issues that have stumped me for years. This new energy and clarity come at an opportune time, for my life has grown much more challenging on two fronts.

First is work. Much of my money I make by parking cars at a couple busy European airports. But if people can't fly, they can't park. When a monster Icelandic volcano grounds European Air Traffic Control, I'm in trouble. Just before the eruption, I'd agreed to invest millions of bucks, borrowing most of it from a Polish bank. Plus, the cessation of flights doesn't put a stop to my day-to-day financial obligations (e.g., payroll, electricity, ash removal), just the revenue to cover them. No one knows when the flights will resume, but everyone thinks this volcano is just the first of many.

Second, on top of this crisis abroad, the lava begins to flow on the home front, too. By now, having fled the Florida condo I'd once finagled them into, my eighty-four-year-old parents are back full time in the D.C. area, ensconced in America's best-equipped, most opulent senior independent-living community. At first, my three siblings and I breathe a collective sigh of relief that our folks are so well attended to, as reflected in a *New York Times* article where my dad says "living at Fox Hill is like living at the Ritz-Carlton." However, in no time my parents are spending less time in the Ritz than they are in the ER.

This shouldn't surprise me, of course. My folks aren't spring chickens. But, still, I'm unprepared for the relentless drumbeat of their health woes. Whenever my cell phone rings, I jump, fretting that it's Mom or Dad, about to relate some new injury, illness, or infection. I want to be there for them, but as a companion caregiver I know my limits. They don't need me so much as they need skilled help.

My anxiety takes on a personal tinge, too, as I worry that my parents' litany is but a trailer for my own Coming Attractions. Mary Jean and Thaddeus Alphonse were both in far better shape when my age (fifty-two). My dad's eyes didn't start going kaput until he was in his mid-seventies; mine cratered in my mid-thirties. My mom got one hip replaced when she turned eighty; I got both replaced when I was forty-eight. Moreover, mentally—somewhat scarily—they can still go toe to toe with me; with my memory slipping more and more, I wonder if Alzheimer's is just around the corner, lying in wait. All told, my Coming Attractions aren't at all comely.

As for my folks' current health status, my dad's had a series of mini- and not-so-mini-strokes and suffers from severe macular degeneration and a variety of chronic infections. He still can't hear much of what's being said (even with his pricey new aural aid), and hunks of his skin get hacked off regularly, his fair complexion reaping what the sun's sown in seven decades of playing golf.

But Tad's mood never flags. He puts on a brave face, for his main concern is Mary Jean. She has more than her own share of chronic health issues, including a mysterious ailment perhaps picked up in Portugal. Also, though my dad still has a number of spry friends and golfing buddies, most of my mom's friends have passed.

I try to help out. I love spending time with my folks. We lunch often, talk regularly over the phone, and swap e-mails. My wife and I invite them to dine with our friends, say, when my business partners visit from London. Everyone loves Mary Jean and Tad.

One afternoon, after a long day of battling more bad news on the Icelandic volcano front, I'm running late for a dinner my wife and I had arranged at Fox Hill. We'd wanted my folks to meet some of our friends who were as close to their age as to ours. But I've hit a glitch.

From my car, I ring Sam Stopak, the main doc handling my eyes. "Sam, I'm running behind. Got started late, then hit terrible traffic on sixty-six. I'm really sorry. You there yet?"

"Just got here."

"Bill and Miriam there?"

"Yes. They were already here when I arrived."

"So, everyone's there except the host and hostess!"

"Well, umm . . ." Sam is truly brilliant, but here his voice takes on the apologetic, befuddled tone he's used so often when peering into my problematic eyes. "Sort of."

"Sort of?"

"Well, upon entering, I passed your parents. Heading out."

"Heading out?"

"Your mom was on a stretcher. An ambulance was taking her to the hospital."

"Oh, my gosh! What's wrong? How'd she look?"

"Well, I'm not an internist, but she looked okay, I guess. I asked your dad, and he said it was just precautionary. Your mom just wasn't feeling well. He told us that he and your mom wanted—*insisted* was the word he used—that we still have our dinner despite their absence."

And so we dine: two doctors, sworn to do no harm; one attorney, sworn to uphold justice; and our spouses, complicit by association. Though we all worry about my mom, we can't help but laugh as well at what we imagine the Fox Hill waitstaff are whispering behind our backs as we heartlessly down our cocktails and ring up the charges on her tab—as she's being rushed to Suburban Hospital's Emergency Room.


## JANUARY 20, 2011

By now, Rosalie's left Haymarket Hospice. While transferring her terrific skill set to another needy charity, she's still helping out part time to ease the transition. Rosalie's replacement as volunteer-services coordinator is Mara Forsten, who, not long after my absurdist dinner party, calls me, asking if I might be able to fill in and visit a guy named Howard Cooper, "just this afternoon . . . just this once."

Mara has been a good student, and she's cagey. Every one of the patients Rosalie assigned me was, supposedly, "short-term." Yet with the exception of my one day with Gordon Ford, my assignments have been averaging more than a year.

I'm not complaining. Quite the opposite. I'll be forever grateful to Rosalie (via Joy, under the auspices of Haymarket Hospice) for conferring upon me the "privilege" (her word, and so fitting) of being able to spend so much time with so many remarkable people.

However, I took loads of statistics courses at George Washington University, the University of Southampton (UK), and the University of Chicago. (I did okay in them.) One of the sins of statistics is confusing association with causation, while a virtue is proper sampling technique, including size. My patients have been handpicked by Rosalie, as opposed to being assigned per a double-blind protocol. Hence, I fully realize that my results being so at variance with NHPCO's industry-wide statistics—most notably a sixty-nine-day mean "length of service," and just 11.4 percent of patients lasting 180 days—is likely just a spurious illustration of Mark Twain's quip "There are lies, damn lies, and statistics."

As I agree with Twain, I seriously doubt I've been part of the "cause" of my patients living longer. But I also agree with Napoleon, who said, "I'd rather be lucky than smart." I've certainly been lucky in whom Rosalie's assigned me. Will Mara keep my lucky streak alive?

Moreover, despite "my" impressive statistics regarding longevity and length of service, one datum has eluded me, the Holy Grail of hospice: The Live Discharge. Nearly one in six patients admitted to hospice are discharged alive. While most are transferred to a more acute-care setting (e.g., Ellen Hensley, from Haymarket Hospice's at-home care, to the ICU at Prince William County Hospital), thousands—annually—are mainstreamed . . . to go on living years, sometimes decades. I want me a Live Discharge . . .

Mara insists this really is a one-time shot. "Mr. Cooper has a regular hospice companion. But a conflict's developed. Plus, Mr. Cooper's daughter is down in Charlottesville, undergoing a round of chemo."

"The daughter?" I say.

"The daughter."

"Cancer?"

"Yes. Cricket lives with him, and she's got it bad."

"That's the daughter's name? Cricket?"

"Yes."

"Who's their nurse?"

"Maureen."

"Yeah!"

"But just his nurse. Not Cricket's."

"Cricket's not involved with hospice?"

"She wants nothing to do with hospice. I mean, as far as she's concerned. As far as she's concerned, she's doesn't need it. She doesn't agree with her doctor's diagnosis."

"Which is?"

"Maureen says it's neck and neck as to who'll go first, Howard or Cricket."

There goes the prospect of my Live Discharge . . . "Man! But, Mara . . . she . . . this . . . Cricket . . . she's the one who asked for some help?"

My question is loaded, double-barreled. First, Mara and I both recall how it was Jim Burris who'd asked for a volunteer. So I wonder if I'll run into any headwinds here with Mr. Cooper, as I did with Little One. Second, when I went off the Reservation and filled those meds for my Mono friend, it was Mara who reprimanded me. Since then, the Haymarket Hospice volunteer-services coordinator and I have only exchanged brief, business-like e-mails.

"The daughter asked, yes. But you'll not face any resistance here. Promise. Unlike with Mrs. Burris, Mr. Cooper's had a hospice companion for some time. Sam Cera. Mr. Cooper is completely on board with your coming by."

"You told him already that I might?"

"Not him. I told Cricket. That you might. I made no guarantees. Just told her I knew of someone who might be able to lend a hand."

As Mara sounds like a reasonable person, a good-hearted person, I feel like I want to clear the air. "Listen, Mara, I wanna say something . . ."

"Please! Let me say something, first?"

"Okay. Sure. If you'd prefer."

"I really hated having to call you, Eric. That Mary Louise business, I mean."

"I could tell."

"But I had to."

"No hard feelings on this end. I totally understand. I'm a lawyer, remember?"

"Yeah. I know. That's, partly, what threw some of us for a loop."

"It was a judgment call. Given the same circumstances, would I do it again? I'm not sure. I certainly *tried* to do the 'right thing.' But I totally see how and why it set off some alarm bells. I just hope it didn't cause any problems for you."

"None at all, but I appreciate your sensitivity."

"So, as regards to today, can you brief me on what's in store?"

"Happy to." What's in store, Mara tells me, is a man with an amalgam of health problems, the biggest being the two balloons inserted beside his heart. If either one pops, he's a goner. "Either could go, any day," says Mara. "Or he could hang on for years."

Howard sounds a lot like my dad. They're both eighty-four, married fifty-plus years, though Howard's wife died in 2000. Both have four kids, though Howard's only son died just months before I enter the picture. Thaddeus has eleven grandchildren to Howard's seven. Both spent time in the Pacific theatre in the mid-40s, though their postings were quite different: Howard was in the Navy, building and installing critical stuff with the Seabees to assist in the invasion of Japan, while Tad was part of the Army occupation force, his scratch golf handicap getting him pressed into service whenever some hack general wanted to win a buck or two from an admiral on Emperor Hirohito's magnificent Mt. Fuji golf course. Both Tad and Howard have iffy hearts and awful eyes and have suffered strokes. One big way they differ is that my dad's worked just two jobs for more than fifty years (parking, developing real estate), whereas Howard's worked twenty-eight different jobs.

"To top it all off," says Mara, "Howard has COPD, kidney failure, and diabetes."

"And a daughter with terminal cancer," I note.

"Right. I guess that's what really tops it all off, isn't it?"

"Sure, Mara, I'll pop on over. But I'm afraid I can't swing four hours. Not today, on such short notice. Sorry. But if I move some things around, I can maybe do two. Would that help?"

"Two'd be great."

"Could I ask you please to call the Coopers and let them know I'll swing by sometime within that four-hour window and that I'll try to stay two hours, give or take?"

"I'll call Cricket right now. Thanks again, Eric. So much."

"Thank you, Mara. If you're anything at all like Rosalie, and it sure sounds like you are, then I know what great, selfless work you're doing. I only see a handful of cases, compared to the hundreds you see. I don't know how you do it, honestly. I don't know how Rosalie did it. I don't know how Joy does it. You ladies are made of much tougher stuff than me."

"That's so kind of you to say. But I'm not tough at all. Just goofy. Some say flat-out insane."

"That's even better! We've gotta grab lunch!"

"Maybe after you visit Mr. Cooper?"

"Deal."

I promptly adjust my schedule, then promptly get lost. By the time I enter "Marsh Run, A Manufactured Home Community," locate Howard's cul-de-sac, park, and hustle up the wooden ramp to his single-wide, I'm fifty minutes late, which leaves me with just seventy minutes before running up against a firm commitment. It hardly seems worth the trip, especially since he'd asked for 240 minutes.

At the end of the ramp, a note's taped to a screen door above a Native American dream catcher, affixed with twine to the bent aluminum handle. As I read *Come on in. —Cricket*, my mind imagines my favorite Native American, Little One, looking down, smiling, a Manhattan in one hand, a cigarette in the other.

I push open the screen door and take a look around. It's dark, so it takes my eyes some time to adjust. When I locate Howard, it's clear from his body language that he's been wondering what the hell happened to me. "I'm so sorry I'm late!" I say as I walk over to shake his hand. "Mr. Cooper, a real pleasure meeting you. I—"

He silences me with a wave—abrupt, yet not at all rude. Just a firm dismissal of my need to issue any sort of apology. "Howard Cooper," he says. Once he's switched on the lamp atop the table beside him and I see his extended hand, I shake it. "Eric Lindner," I respond.

His smile's easy, his handshake hearty. He's got the same complexion as my mom and Little One: light mocha. He's seated in a chair, in a nook by a window, surrounded by the usual hospice paraphernalia: a stand of oxygen tanks resembling World War II howitzer shells, a motorized wheelchair, a magnifying glass. But I see less typical stuff, too: a tape recorder, a tin of chewing tobacco, a pair of crinkled Western boots. "Have a seat," he says, indicating his wheelchair.

Though I feel a bit odd doing so, I sit. "Those are some interesting-looking boots."

After a slight adjustment to the breathing prongs stuck up his nose, he comes to life, like I've plunked a nickel into a nineteenth-century Coney Island mechanical fortune teller. He reaches down beside his chair, stretching the sleeve of his T-shirt, causing an upper-arm tattoo to peek out: a horse head, faded with time and atrophy. He takes a deep, labored, breath, fighting through the viscous phlegm occasioned by his chronic obstructive pulmonary disease. "G-g-got 'em in Montana. F-f-forty-seven. *Hrrack!*" He lifts up a small wastebasket, hocks into it, lowers it back to the floor, reaches for a tissue, wipes his lips, tosses this into the trash, grabs his boots, and hands them to me. His pride is palpable. The boots clearly hold special meaning.

I run my fingers along the blue leather, fancy scrolling, and silver studs before flicking the iron rowels. "They're nice. Much nicer than the ones my son got in Montana when he and I were out there a few months back. We got ours at Boot Barn. These gotta be custom."

He nods. "S-s-seventy-nine dollars. Pretty much all what I s-saved up as a Seabee during the war. 'Course, I'd a saved a heck of a lot more if'n I'd not while on shore leave spent so much at bars, in honky-tonks, and on . . . other things."

"Still," I say to Howard, "seventy-nine bucks? In forty-seven?? That sounds rich. And, what a memory! Most days I can't remember what I had for breakfast."

He shakes his head. "A-average. Good ones'd cost twice that much. *Hrrack!*"

"You like horses, I guess." I wag my head at his left arm, site of the equine tattoo.

He nods.

"Born in Montana, Mr. Cooper?"

He shakes his head. "Virginia. Browntown. Near F-F-Front Royal. *Hr-hr-hrrack!*" A coughing fit occupies him for a good twenty seconds. Again he retrieves the waste basket and expectorates. "Excuse me."

"No need to apologize. Gosh. What took you to Montana, then?"

From his face I infer an answer: adventure. He smiles wanly, like a once-avid but now out-of-practice storyteller. These days, given his depleted ticker, bad eyes, and weak lungs, he's mostly consigned to listening to stories. He reaches for his chaw: Skoal.

Given Howard's precarious health, the last thing he should be doing is "dipping," but he doesn't seem to care. While it may make it a little harder to talk, and breathe—some nicotine shrapnel perhaps even popping one of his arterial balloons, killing him—chewing tobacco makes life more livable. The chaw is grist for his memory mill, transporting him back to when he was a Seabee, laying pontoons in Okinawa, a cowboy, branding steers in South Dakota, a young buck, skinny dipping with the teen-age beauties up and around Browntown. The returns are worth the risk.

As methodically as a sommelier uncorking a $10,000 bottle of Chateau whatever, Howard unscrews the tin lid, pinches a small clump of moist, aromatic Kentucky steel cut, and tucks it between his cheek and gum. "W-w-working at the stables, in Front Royal . . ." Hearing me sniffle, he hands me a box of Kleenex. Seeing me fumble the handoff, he pushes the lamp closer to me so I can see better.

"Thanks." I blow my nose. The viscous honk brings a smile to his face. "You mean, Mr. Cooper, along five twenty-two, up over Chester Gap?"

Howard's flashing eyes suggest surprise—and delight—at my knowing such trivia. The stables were shuttered sixty years ago. The place is now a wildlife preserve run by the National Zoo, where they breed rare Yukon lynx and track poacher-endangered, chip-implanted elephants as they sip and sup in the Serengeti.

"Only reason I know this," I explain, "is that a friend of mine—ninety-year-old Elmer Hensley, born up in Haymarket—used horses from those very stables when he was a member of the Coast Guard's Beach Patrol, during World War Two."

"Ahh . . ." He nods, and holds out the trashcan, into which I deposit my snotty tissue. "Thank you, sir. Elmer trotted up and down the coast, down 'round Hampton Roads."

"U.S. Army stables," Howard says. "C-c-cavalry. Where Teddy Roosevelt's Rough Riders trained." Before lowering the can to the floor, he spits into it for good measure.

"The days of cavalry charges," say I, "ended with Hitler's Panzer tanks, though."

"Didn't run across that fella. S-served in the Pacific. Plenty busy there, though."

"Same's Elmer. I'll have to get you guys together."

Howard grabs another tissue and pats some sputum that's stubbornly clinging to his chin and lips. He balls up the waste and drops it into the can, now on the floor.

"Tell me a bit about Montana, will you? Unless, of course, it's too uncomfortable for you to talk."

"W-well now . . . when I get out the Navy, weren't no jobs. But I had a friend who had a friend who knew a man . . . had two ranches. In C-C-Colorado, South Dakota. So . . ."

I'm transfixed. Time flies. I lose track of it. Glancing at my cell phone, I see I'm way late for my next appointment, a key meeting to discuss the progress (or lack thereof) regarding the major renovations at Gdańsk airport, which have a critical bearing on my financial well-being. But as parking in Poland is so much less fascinating and entertaining than what I'm here doing I hold up my phone. "Pardon me?"

"You go right ahead."

"Thanks." I tap out a text. *Held up. Go on wo me. Will conf in later.*

But I don't conference in later, because I don't want this to be my one and only visit. Even though my schedule is packed, family and work problematic, my gut tells me I've got to find time for this man, that there's something in store for me here that I've not found elsewhere with my other patients (special though they've all been).

Once he's finished telling me about his time as a ranch hand, I ask, "When does your regular volunteer visit?"

"Tuesdays and Thursdays. T-ten to two. Sam Cera's his name."

"What's Sam do when he visits?"

"He—*hrrack*! . . . r-r-reads to me."

"What's he read?"

"Will James. Or . . . the Bible."

"Never heard of Will James."

"He w-w-wrote back in the fifties. W-W-Westerns."

"So you like Westerns, huh?"

He eyes me, nods toward his boots, then rolls up his sleeve, exposing his stallion.

"Dumb question!"

He smiles.

"And the Bible? Want me to read the Bible?"

His facial expression doesn't quite say *Dumb question*. More like *Thanks, but no thanks*.

I think for a minute. "Okay. Ever heard of *Lonesome Dove*?"

"Think I s-s-saw it on TV. While ago."

"Yeah. The book came out in nineteen eighty or so. The TV miniseries didn't do much for me, but I loved the novel. It won the Pulitzer Prize. Want me to bring it along next time, see if you like it?"

"That sounds real g-g-good. Thank you."

"Okay then. We've got a plan. I'm not sure when I'll next be able to swing by, but I'm already looking forward to it. And when I do, we'll take *Lonesome Dove* out for a trot."

"I s-s-sure 'preciate it, Eric."

"My pleasure, Mr. Cooper."

After we shake hands, while I'm gathering up my things, I reflect for a moment on the protocol regarding how we should address each other. Do we use first names or Mr. This and That? For me it's always a matter of applying common sense, of not being presumptuous, of being a bit more Polish, in that sometimes Poles who've known each other for years still address each other as Sir or Madam. Eventually it becomes clear what each party prefers. But there can be awkwardness. For instance, early on I felt comfortable calling Gordon Ford's widow Dorothy, yet though I've asked her many times to please call me Eric, I've stopped doing so, for she prefers Mr. Lindner or when talking about me over the phone, in my presence, the hospice man. Here the implicit protocol is, He'll call me Eric, I'll call him Mr. Cooper.

The moment I pull out of his driveway, I start noodling over how—not whether—I'm going to reorganize my schedule to see more of Howard.

During my drive home, I'm again struck by the paradox of serving as a volunteer. I'm supposed to be the giver here, providing companionship for this lonely dude. Yet even after only one visit I already feel like I'm on the receiving end of a big gift—a special windfall in the form of a special relationship. This paradox is reported all the time by volunteers. My initial report includes the following excerpt:

> Filled in for S. Cera—got acquainted.
> What a great man!! Very sad!

Over the next few days, I make some inquiries. Joy gushes, "Isn't Mr. Cooper amazing? But," she adds, "watch out for Cricket! I asked her if she wanted a companion, too. Just trying to help, you know? And she nearly bit my head off! '*I'm not ready to die!*' she yelled, over the phone. Nearly broke my eardrum. Then, after simmering down a bit, she added, 'Quitting's not in my vocabulary!'"

Maureen adds to what she told me prior to my initial visit. "This one's hard for me. Really hard. He could go any day. He's such a lovely man."

But it's Mara who closes the sale, once we grab lunch at a Thai restaurant. It's our first time meeting, and we hit it off right away. She reminds me of Joy, what with her short, wavy, light-colored hair and seemingly caffeinated, definitely discursive demeanor. And though her attire is comparably casual, Mara's eyes are worse (she wears glasses). Just as easygoing as Joy, Mara is also hilarious. Equal parts Lucille Ball and Mother Teresa, she's got that dry, piercing Midwestern wit that I so loved when living in Chicago. Mara totally gets the alchemy of hospice: how laugh-out-loud comedy and crushing sadness can coexist in poignant equipoise. She gets it because she's been through it, having been told that her one-year-old son had a brain tumor so he'd not live long, yet he lived to be nineteen. "Funny thing was, one of the best parts of that whole experience was what my dad said to me, afterward: 'Mara, I'm really proud of how you handled yourself through all this.' Man! I sure could have used a lot more of that growing up! It made me realize: we've got to seize every rare and wonderful experience we run across—no matter the source. I think you've got yourself one . . . in Howard Cooper. I'd seize it."

Helga tells me more about Cricket, too. The daughter doesn't like leaving Howard alone when she's seeing her own doctors, undergoing chemo and radiation, or rummaging through the recent arrivals at the local food bank.

Cricket's a case study in thrift, illustrating how much one can accomplish on a shoestring budget. In addition to Haymarket Hospice staff and volunteers, she's enlisted another dozen to help her dad, free of charge, ranging from Howard's heart, ear, and eye doctors at a West Virginia Veteran's Administration Hospital to (1) the sheet-metalworker who manufactures in and then drives from Ohio to install a custom ramp, (2) the V.A. guy who cleans the mobile home twice a week, and (3) the neighbor who mows the Coopers' thin strip of lawn.

## JANUARY 23

While at home, gathering my Kindle and stuff, preparing to head over for my second visit, I reach for my favorite new cap. (For reasons of eye safety and light sensitivity, I almost always wear a cap. I got this one several months earlier when in Montana with my son.) It's beat-to-hell denim, the kind of thing most guys love but makes their wives cringe. On its front, in faded red letters, it reads *Bull Riding*. It's immediately clear that this cowboy headgear was intended not for me but for Howard, to facilitate his reminiscing about the days when he in fact rode bulls. My wife hates this cap. She'd be delighted were I to fob it off to Howard.

Now in the Western genre, my thoughts turn to another aspect of Howard's erstwhile ensemble: his boots. Though Howard can no longer walk, I figure a pair of my boots will do him more good than me, so I hustle up to my eBay-culled barn (where I'd found Gordon's horse book and Elmer's Jesus bullet), root around a bit, and find this custom set, made from a nineteen-foot African python a friend had given me. Tucked inside one boot is the matching belt I had made.

I arrive to find Howard sitting in his chair. Though blind, he's looking out the window, smiling. He doesn't notice me. But I notice him. His

countenance suggests he's deriving far more true joy from the warm sun
and faint breeze filtering into his mobile home than some Russian baux-
ite billionaire who one second before christening his football field–sized
yacht learns from his favorite catamite's whisper that the day before his
hated peer tin oligarch had christened a vessel one inch longer than his
own seagoing phallic symbol.

It's a bright day. The sun's rays partly illuminate the dark interior,
but I need to watch my step because the 288-square-foot trailer (32 feet
by 9) is a mob scene. Perhaps I hadn't noticed it during my first visit
because Cricket was out. But I do today, for it's hard not tripping or
banging into something. In addition to three humans, there's

- a small dog with a satellite-dish prophylaxis, and a gargantuan
  teddy bear;
- a sofa, two easy chairs, a jammed bathroom, a fully equipped
  kitchen (including a dinette set, complete with four chairs), and
  two fully furnished bedrooms;
- Mr. Cooper's wheelchair, oxygen tanks, and a stack of cassette
  tapes on the floor (histories of China, the Second Amendment),
  attesting to his range of interest and caliber of intellect;
- at least a dozen yard gnomes, a half-dozen other stuffed animals,
  and scores of snow globes and other tchotchkes, lining the shelves
  and cluttering the floor;
- various types of guns and ammo, along with sheaves of shot-to-hell
  paper targets;
- a Sputnik-era TV that looks like it's never been used;
- a big Bible, laying open, on a stand, like in a library; and
- Jesus, along with his disciples, in a dark print of Da Vinci's *Last
  Supper*.

Cricket's asleep on the sofa. She's slight, well shy of five feet tall, but
behind her, as both pillow and protector, burly arms wrapped around
her small shoulders, is the biggest teddy bear I've ever seen. It's twice
her size.

A bark awakens Cricket. "Oh . . . hello," she says to me, groggily,
pointing at the shaggy yellow mutt, collared with one of those bizarre

plastic snow-cone-shaped contraptions designed, I think, to keep the dog from cannibalizing itself. "That's Huggy. Bad dog. Waking me up." Cricket cocks her thumb at the massive bear. "And this is Teddy." She returns her head to Teddy's chest and tries to go back to sleep.

"Why hello!" says Howard, Huggy's bark having shattered his reverie.

"Hi, Mr. Cooper."

"See you met Crick."

"I did. And Teddy. And Huggy."

Maureen's told me Cricket takes Teddy just about everywhere— "short of the shower and the toilet. She takes that thing to doctor's appointments, the gas station, the gun range, Wal-Mart." Beside the front door hangs a framed certificate. Awarded to "Cricket Cooper" by the Cancer Centers of America, it signifies that she's completed a round of treatment. Beside Cricket's certificate is another, awarded to "Teddy Cooper." He completed a round, too.

As if to apologize for his daughter's tuning me out, Howard says "Crick's tired. H-h-have a seat." Though a second lounge chair's not too far away nor the dinette chairs, as before he wants me to sit in his wheelchair.

So I do. "The engine turned off?"

He laughs as he clicks the switch on the end-table lamp then slides his hand down and over for his tin of chewing tobacco.

I present him with my goodie bag. "What's this?" he says. He peers inside the bag but then goes for his magnifying glass. He retrieves the cap and brings it up close to his face. Like my dad, he suffers from advanced macular degeneration, so I know how Howard needs to move his head back and forth and around, piecing together the fragmented, pin-holed remnants of vision. "B-Bull . . . Ri . . . ding . . . ? Bull Riding??"

"You got it! It's yours, Mr. Cooper."

He frowns the frown of a man with an intense, innate dislike of being on the receiving end of charity. (His being the main beneficiary of Cricket's less-inhibiting compunctions notwithstanding.) A man used to eating only what he kills. A man who's never had a credit card, never used an ATM, but can trap, dress, and cook just about anything that one can hook or bag in the rivers and wilds of Virginia.

"Please take it?" I plead. "Otherwise, my wife'll just throw it out. "

His frown gives way to a wheezy laugh.

"See . . . if you wear it, at least I'll enjoy seeing it a little, from time to time."

He places the cap on his head, reaches back into the bag, yanks out one of my exotic python boots, and draws it close to his face. He rubs the scaly, slick, black-and-brown snakeskin, inspects the heel, the boot tip, the pulls. "These are s-s-something . . ."

I grab the matching belt from the other boot and hand it to him. "My Ethiopian friend gave me this really long skin some twenty years ago, but it took me a decade before I could find a guy to make me a pair of custom boots. Not as many boot makers around these days as there were when you were a cowboy, Mr. Cooper. Thought I'd have no problem finding someone near me, given all the riders and farmers. But there aren't any, not a one. The guy who made these? His shop's in Brooklyn, New York." (My thoughts flit to Dolly, before returning to Howard.) "Guy had a booth at the Washington International Horse Show. That's how I got hold of him. Think he did a pretty good job, don't you?"

"R-really good."

"You can keep 'em if you like. I don't wear 'em that often."

"I c-c-can't accept these. But thank you." He hands me back my boot.

I set the pair on the floor, beside Huggy, who hauls herself and her plastic prophylaxis over to investigate the foreign object and its alien smells. "So . . . I've downloaded *Lonesome Dove* on my Kindle." I raise the device. "How 'bout we give it a try?"

"Sounds good."

"All right, then, let's say we head back out West, shall we?"

He's pumped. I can tell by the smile creasing his face, the twinkle piercing his macular morass, the wad of tobacco plumping his cheek, and how he's settling back into his easy chair, tugging and adjusting the Bull Riding cap. The sense I get is, he's back in South Dakota, in '47, penned in, atop an ornery, longhorn-swinging bull, having just given the thumbs-up to the rodeo master to open the gate . . . to the roar of the crowd, the delight of the ladies, and the envy of all the other cowboys who didn't have the balls to mount and ride the fearsome beast . . .

As if she can sense some excitement and doesn't want to miss out, Cricket yawns, stretches her arms, and rolls her head away from the window, toward us.

"Join us, Crick," says Howard.

I turn, wave, and, taking note of the nearly obliterated gun-range target beside her head, say, "Not much left of that target. What'd you use?"

"Everything I got. Dan Wesson forty-four mag, long barrel. Sig Sauer three-eighty. Glock thirty-two." She goes on to explain how all the caregivers she's requisitioned represent but a part of her strategy for homeland defense. She always leaves Howard with her Sig Sauer. "It's under his chair. Daddy don't need to see to double-tap some punk who's stupid enough to barge in and try to rob him while I'm out. But it wouldn't be no one from around here, as everyone around here knows Daddy's reputation."

"You sure seem to know your guns."

"Ought to. Daddy taught me. Best shot in the County. 'Fore his eyes gave out." Cricket tells me how she sleeps on the .380. "The thirty-two I pack in my purse. If I overnight anywhere, like in Charlottesville, to see my doctor? I bring Dan."

"How big is Dan?"

"Weighs in at five pounds. What being a long barrel, he hardly fits in my laptop case."

"You carry around a five-pound gun with you a lot?"

"Sure. I'm not taking any chances. But . . . you go on and read to Daddy. We'll talk later." Cricket rolls back over toward the window.

After an hour or so of reading, I say, "I get the feeling you like it, Mr. Cooper."

"Surely do."

"Great, then," I say, as I stand, preparing to shove off. "So we've got a plan. This book's a big one, almost nine hundred pages. So we'll be out West together for some time."

He pinches the bill of his Bull Riding cap. "Thank you kindly. I look forward to it. Thank you for c-c-coming by."

"See you next time, then. And . . . bye, Cricket."

"Eric?" she says, still not facing me.

"Yes?

"If it's not too much trouble, when you come by next time, could you maybe bring me a frappé from McDonald's?"

"Sure, Cricket. What type?"

"Mocha."

"Nothing for Teddy?"

She laughs. Now she rolls over to look me squarely in the eye. "Teddy can do a lot. He's the Teddy Roosevelt of teddy bears. Written a hundred thirty-five pages of my biography. Already arranged my funeral. Gonna be one helluva time! Teddy'll be the bouncer. Gonna need one! With my kin, things're bound to get out of hand! My sister, now there's a piece of work! But Teddy can't sip no frappé."

## FEBRUARY 18

Despite seven visits and five frappés, Cricket remains a bit stand-offish, guarded. What breaks the ice between us is the tale of my brief—fool-hardy—stint as a matador. In *Lonesome Dove* at the moment, a pint-sized, irascible old bull by the name of Old Red, seemingly intent on committing suicide, is stomping and snorting, about to charge a huge, ferocious grizzly bear, which prompts me to shut my Kindle and spin my own tale of testosterone run amok. "So I'm in Avila, Spain, with this German friend, visiting this place where they breed and train bulls before shipping them off to the big cities?"

Howard straightens up in his seat. A happy cough blasts through some phlegm.

"I'll be honest, I've had a few beers . . ."

"Ha!" he exclaims.

"Right!" adds Cricket. "A few. How old were you?"

"Twenty-one," I say.

"So," she stipulates, sounding like the paralegal she was hoping and training to be, "for the record, old enough to know better."

"So I've been told."

Howard slaps his thigh.

"So," Cricket asks, "what happens?"

"Well, you know how matadors wave 'round those red capes? Well, they're useless."

"The bulls are color blind," she says.

"That's right, Cricket. You ever fought a bull?"

"No. Fought plenty of jackasses. But never a bull."

"C-c-crick!" says her dad, for once thrilled at the detour from fiction to real life.

"Nice," I say, eyeing her. "Anyway, so my German friend and his coconspirator, this even more boozed-up ex-matador bull trainer, goad my ego and dare me to step into the ring to take on this bull. It's not in the ring yet, see, but they assure me it'll be, well, about as big and ferocious as Huggy."

At the mention of her name, Huggy stops sniffing a Gnome's crotch, tilts her head, and wags her tail, rattling her ridiculous headgear.

"I seen this movie before," says Cricket.

"I'll tell you something, it isn't easy not moving—hauling off in the opposite direction, to be precise—when eight hundred pounds of Pissed Off comes charging at you."

Howard's eyes flash in kinship. He's laughing so hard he fumbles then drops his tin of chewing tobacco. "B-been there, d-done that . . ."

"Then you get the picture, Mr. Cooper."

Cricket hands Howard his tobacco. "So?" she says. "What happens?"

I lift my jeans. "See that?" My index finger taps an ankle scar, about four inches long.

Her fingers tug down the corners of her mouth, caricaturing a pout. "Poor Eric got a boo-boo! That's nothing! You don't want to get into a scar duel with me, 'cause you'll lose. Badly.

"Or me," mumbles Howard, his mouth packed with chaw.

"So, you moved?" she says. She shakes her head, disdainfully. "Well, at least you were smart enough to take anesthesia before your biopsy."

"For the record," I say, "I want to make it clear that once I'd leapt out the ring? And recouped my manly, American pride? I get right back in there for a second go. This time, I stand stock still as the beast whooshes right past me. I'll tell you, now that was a thrill."

While driving home, I think about how glad I am that my idiotic tempting of fate can provide some enjoyment, for though Howard isn't tempting fate, it's wreaking havoc nonetheless. His son's just died. His daughter's health is dire. He could go any day. My report reflects my awe and admiration:

> Yet, thru it all, he's as warm and lovely and noncomplaining as anyone I've ever met in my life.

## FEBRUARY 21

Howard's laid up in Fauquier Hospital, pursuant to another COPD attack. As he looks distracted, wistful, I wonder if he's reminded of some
previous visit with his wife, Florence. He's never uttered her name in
my presence, but from Cricket I know that his bride's death devastated
him. Flo was his devoted sidekick, wet and dry. They'd spent more than
their fair share of time in hospitals, having babies, stitching up wounds,
sobering up.

When Cricket mentions that Lee Lund is on the way over, Howard's
mood transforms—instantly. He fiddles with the bed controls so he's sitting up, so as to look less invalid. Blind and bedridden, he still does what
he can to tidy up his immediate vicinity, including brushing his hair, the
first and only time I see him do so.

"Howard!" Lee purrs, as she enters his hospital room and slinks
up beside him. She's tall, lanky, sensual—and knows it. Something
about her rekindles the old flame. That the Haymarket Hospice social
worker is four decades younger than him just piques his interest more.
Furthermore, he's not at all inhibited about flirting in the presence of
his daughter.

This is my cue to skedaddle. "You've now got much more interesting company, Howard. So I'll see you later." He completely ignores my
departure. I couldn't be happier.

After a few days, Howard is released.

But he returns a few weeks later for an operation on his esophagus.
Entering his hospital room, I see Cricket in the corner, smoking. Alert
to the possibility of a nurse coming through the door, she's strategically
positioned to dispose of the evidence out the window.

I point at her. "Busted."

After a final drag, she flicks the butt out the window and exhales.
"Nazis."

"How'd the operation go?"

"Good. Daddy'll be able to talk more with less pain. At least that's
what the docs think, anyway."

"And, Cricket, how are things with you?"

Howard opens his eyes.

She wheels on him. "Don't you dare try to speak, Daddy!"

"You might want to just rest, Mr. Cooper. But nod if you want me to read." He nods, so I return to Larry McMurtry's masterpiece.

## FEBRUARY 26

Cricket appears to be warming up to me a bit. Or at least Teddy is, judging from the following e-mail, which I receive in response to one I sent while overseas, on a business trip:

Dearest Eric:

Ths "TEDDY"! U bee crfull n forin cntry.

Wtch u bk.

## MARCH 1

I can tell right off that something's not right. Howard's awake, he sees me, but he says nothing. He continues staring out the window. Normally, his welcome is over the top.

Cricket approaches. "Daddy's busted up. My uncle's just died of a heart attack . . ."

Howard turns my way. "Hello, Eric." Now I understand why this extremely proud and polite man has been ignoring me. He'd wanted to wipe away his tears. But the Seabee did an imperfect job of swabbing his cheeks, for the tracks are evident, glistening in the bright sun that streaks through the window.

"Hey, Mr. Cooper. I . . . I really don't know what to say about your brother . . . other than to tell you how deeply sorry I am for your loss."

I rest a hand on his shoulder, but he doesn't respond. "Up for some reading?" I say. "Sure," he responds. But his flat tone suggests he's just being polite; seeing how I drove all the way out to see him, he figures it'd be rude to send me packing.

One of the many things I love about my Kindle is how it always opens up to where I've left off. But such techno-wizardry is superfluous in

Howard's case. He always remembers where we left off and enjoys telling me before my Kindle does. "Hell Bitch," he says, as I open to where this horse is getting her jollies jettisoning *Lonesome Dove* heroes in between biting off hunks of their flesh. I'm prompted to ask, "You ever get bucked?"

"More t-t-times than I can remember." The recollection brings a smile to his face.

"Was it painful or just embarrassing?"

"Only a been embarrassing if'n I'd a not hopped right back up onto my own hell bitch. You understand. I can tell. That's why you did what you did over in Spain. And that's how I've always approached life, too. Not worrying about being embarrassed. Worrying about getting embarrassed drains all the fun out of life."

"You're a wise man, Mr. Cooper. A lucky man." Did I really just say to a man—who hasn't a penny to his name, can't see, walk, breathe, or bathe without help, whose heart might give out any second, a widower who mourns the loss of his beloved every waking hour, who's recently lost his only son, just lost his beloved brother, and whose cherished, cancer-ridden daughter might also die any day—that he's lucky??

Though I know he heard me, Howard's way too polite to acknowledge as much, so he changes the subject. "D-don't understand why there're so many mares."

"What do you mean?"

"Mares don't make good mounts."

"Why not?"

"C-cause they're finicky. Attract st-st-stallions. Estrus."

"That's interesting. So I guess either McMurtry is trying to make some literary point or he doesn't know his horses, like you."

A knock at the door interrupts us.

"Come on in," says Cricket, her angelic voice backed up by the pistol under her butt.

"Aloha," says a man, as he enters, guitar case slung over his shoulder. His salutation seals it: even before he'd opened his mouth, with his mop of half-wavy, half-curly dirty-blond hair, pale blue eyes, Jesus Fish ear-stud, cocoa skin, bleached teeth, and longboard pendant, he'd already looked like a surfer dude from Hanalei Bay, an especially interesting one at that.

"Daddy," Cricket announces for the benefit of her blind father, "it's Chaplain Chris."

This is my first time meeting Chris Black, the Haymarket Hospice chaplain who's replaced the man I met during Bob Zimmerman's "burial mediation," who's since died. Chris has a surfer's body, too: deceptively strong, his chest and arms powerful from swimming and paddling, often against a strong current. His rugged Viking Irish face radiates good cheer. His expansive smile seems 100 percent genuine. He doesn't strike me as a snake-oil salesman. But his arrival does involve an under-tow, judging by the pouting faces of Howard and Cricket.

After introducing myself to Chris and stepping over to shake his hand, I ask Howard, "Want me to stop my reading so Chris here can play some guitar?"

Howard fidgets. He doesn't want to hurt Chris's feelings. This man for whom the possibility of embarrassment provokes no fear isn't about to visit any embarrassment upon his guest. In Howard's Bible, that's a cardinal sin.

"Oh," says Chris, fingering his surfboard pendant, the knot in his frayed leather band snagged by his starboard clavicle. The board flips over, revealing a Celtic cross, once painted gold, but now only the faintest patina remains, the flakes having dissolved and merged into the soft brown tone and erratic grain of what I'd guess to be koa wood. "I didn't mean to interrupt. I can come back if this is a bad time. Should'a called ahead."

"Not at all, Chris," I say. "I was the one who popped by unannounced. I'm the one who should apologize. I was just about to leave. How 'bout if I read for five more minutes, then I'd like to hang around and listen to you play a song. Sound like a plan?" I look to Howard.

He's stifled his pouting. He sighs, falls back into his chair, removes his Bull Riding cap, hangs it on the window latch, and glances down at his boots.

I stop reading just as some Texas horse thieves are about to throw down with some Mexican horse thieves. "That's a good place to stop. Nothing like clear-cut moral ambiguity."

Cricket laughs. Howard slaps his thigh. Chaplain Chris scratches his chin.

I touch Howard's wrist. "I'll pick it up later this week, okay?" I nod at Chris.

"Mahalo!" He's unzipped his case and lain his guitar across his lap before my Kindle's powered down. He strums some strings and fiddles with the tuning knobs. "I'm no Bob Dylan, but I've just written this. Hope you like it. I call it, 'Let's Ride That Big Jesus Wave Together.'"

## MARCH 4

Rarely do I see Howard eat. Every now and then when I arrive he's munching a potato chip. (Sour cream and onion, his favorite.) But he'll roll up the bag and stow it. Cricket says he loves his morning donut (always honey glazed), but I never see him eat a one.

I know he doesn't like prairie chicken, though. After reading a passage in *Lonesome Dove* where this resourceful girl catches and cooks the fowl and this indolent guy expresses surprise and delight at how wonderful it tastes, Howard says, "That's not how I r-remember it."

"Any other food memories of your days as a cowboy?"

He thinks for a moment. "C-coffee."

"Coffee? What about coffee?"

"First time I paid ten cents for a cup of c-c-coffee."

"Was that high or low?"

"Everywhere else, it'd always been just five cents. I thought they were just trying to t-t-take advantage of me, seeing as how I was from Virginia."

"Where'd this outrage take place?"

He laughs. "Oklahoma C-C-City. Greyhound b-b-bus station."

When it's time for me to leave, Cricket grabs her cigarettes and follows me out the door. "Just heading out for a smoke, Daddy."

I step aside to let her pass. The screen door slaps shut. "Got a minute?" she says. "Sure." I brush past the malfunctioning dream catcher and follow her.

Once out back, she flicks away some bird poop and sits on one of two wobbly green plastic Adirondack chairs. I sit beside her. She tries to fire up, but her lighter's being uncooperative. "You now?" A soft whimper escapes as her body shakes. I reach over, gently pry the lighter from her hand, and, after a few flicks, raise a flame. She bends over to the soft sound of paper crackling, takes a deep drag, holds it, then exhales. "My C'ville oncologist showed me the latest X-rays. It's late stage four. It's everywhere, and it's inoperable. I believe him. He's a rare doc. Not a butthead. Can't bring myself to tell Daddy. I don't want to add to his stress. I mean, if he's going soon, why go with an even heavier heart during his final months?"

"I am so, so sorry, Cricket."

She wipes away a tear. "What should I do, Eric? Should I tell him?"

I bite my lip. Cricket has solicited my input, so this isn't an instance of my offering unsolicited advice, one of Rosalie's major *Don'ts*. Still, I'm reluctant to weigh in. "I'd be a liar if I said I had much of an idea. But I can say you're being a very loving daughter in how you're approaching this. How sensitive you're being." I reach over and hug her, trying not to burn my good eye in the process. "You know I'll do whatever I can to help you and your father."

"I know you will. You know . . . there's a reason for everything. A reason Sam Cera couldn't be here that day . . . a reason you were able to step in.

"The only thing I'm worried about is Daddy. This news I've just learned? It'll break his heart. They say just about the hardest thing in life is for a parent to watch his child die. And, 'course, Daddy's just been through this with Howard Junior. Now, his brother up and dies. Daddy's got a strong heart. But nobody's heart is unbreakable."

In between drags, she goes into the history of her cancer: nearly a decade-long ordeal of gut instincts . . . rising to suspicions . . . evolving to missed, mysterious, and often conflicting diagnoses, botched and excruciating biopsies, joyful remission—and then tragic, traumatic relapse. "When the cancer was first suspected, in oh-five, they tell me the biopsy will be a piece of cake. 'You'll hardly notice it,' they say. But it's unbearable. Back then, when I'm ninety-five pounds, it takes three big guys to keep me pinned down. Even with my being supposedly heavily sedated. I'm thrashing about, yelling, screaming, kicking. They were damn lucky none of my pistols was within reach! They used this sadistically long three-pronged grabber to yank out clumps of breast tissue. And the biopsies . . . they were just the beginning."

She endured six months of hell, including a double-mastectomy, preceded by chemo and radiation to reduce what would be removed, followed by additional rounds to try and make the area inhospitable to cancer cells. Also involved were alternating bouts of diarrhea and locked bowels, hair loss, and chronic insomnia. Her goal was to get ahead of the rapidly metastasizing cancer, but her prognosis wasn't good.

However, the worst part of it all wasn't the cutting, the puking, or how her hair cleaved off in clumps while shampooing. Though at the time the cancer was only apparent in one breast, akin to Angelina Jolie's brave, proactive decision, Cricket insisted that both be removed. She spent tons of time surfing the Internet, talking with friends, researching her family's history. Her conclusion: though the X-rays might not yet have detected any evidence of cancer cells in the left breast, the cells were there, lurking, incubating, mobilizing for metastasis. She decided, better scorched earth than no earth at all.

But whenever a patient presses for more extensive surgery than the surgeon recommends, a red flag goes up. So before her oncologist and surgeon would sign off on a double-mastectomy, they insisted Cricket see a shrink. She already had a shrink, but they insisted she see this particular shrink. Five minutes into the session, after mumbling about "puerile proclivities" and Teddy's "obvious Freudian role," the young woman cut to her bizarro chase: "Cricket, you have to accept the important role your breasts play in your womanhood."

Cricket (nearly twice the woman's age) replied, "Excuse me?? My boobs don't make me who I am! I don't need them. I'm not having any more babies. This is my life on the line! My life's not worth pushing up daisies with two knockers.

"In every bad thing that happens, I try to find something good. With the diagnosis of cancer, I figured, if I can't have some fun with it? I'm not going to play along. Besides, Teddy brings out the best in people. Most people, at least. The little kids in the cancer-treatment center just love him to death. Pun intended."

Cricket rose, grabbed her biographer (Teddy), and stormed out. At least she'd left on a high note: her appetite had returned. All the docs had been telling her she had to eat, but what with all the worry, toxins, anesthesia, and fatigue, seldom was she hungry. When she was, it was ephemeral: once she'd ingested some dry toast or bland soup, she felt like upchucking. But the run-in with the shrink had made her ravenous.

The battle with the shrink is ancient history by the time I enter the picture. The way Cricket sees it, acting "puerile" bought her four good years, at least.

But things aren't so good now. Either some of the cells first detected in 2005 were hiding "in the margins" or swimming around at undetectably minute levels in the bloodstream, or some new nuclei hatched to form altogether new cells. Whatever the malignancy's provenance, the cancer's back. Worse than ever.

At least her appetite's better than ever. She can really put it away. Once I bring her a massive Red Truck coffee cake, about as big around and heavy as a manhole cover, and she nearly consumes it in one sitting. "Got a little carried away," she says. "Gave the rest . . . a few crumbs . . . to my neighbor."

## AUGUST 16

I've been traveling tons, yet still I've managed to visit Howard twenty-one times over the past five months. When out of town, I've tried to call every few days, send an e-mail or a postcard.

My typical visit lasts about ninety minutes, on top of a drive of ninety minutes, round-trip. As it is today, my typical routine involves reading *Lonesome Dove*. Thankfully, it's a big book.

Also thankfully, the volcano seems to have been a one-off event. Plus, Poland's on a tear, being the only country in the EU to have avoided recession. This leads a Belgian behemoth to court me, seeing if I might like to sell my company. Now, it's not so much a matter of trying to survive but thrive, either by remaining an entrepreneur, selling, or joint-venturing.

Also thankfully, my parents are quiescent. Their decision to vacate their new Florida villa and return to D.C. full time did create some initial chaos, but things have settled down.

## AUGUST 28

Howard, Cricket, and I spend eight hours together, including four at the big V.A. medical center in Martinsburg, West Virginia. The place is awash with Seabees and other veterans, their caps, T-shirts, and jackets emblazoned with battles fought, proclaiming "Go, Navy!" and whatnot.

Wearing his Bull Riding cap, Howard gets his heart checked, his eyes checked, and his hearing checked.

As we make our way between appointments, as Howard self-propels (he won't let me help), Cricket pushes Teddy around in a wheelchair, prompting all sorts of looks. The adults look perplexed or—for reasons that escape me—peeved, whereas all the kids, reacting as if there's nothing at all out of the ordinary, are elated at the sight of the tiny, ashen-faced lady pushing the big, apparently disabled bear whose NRA T-shirt reads *Support the right to arm bears*.

## SEPTEMBER 12

Howard tells me he took a spill a few days prior. "My legs just gave out. No more bull riding for me, I guess."

Cricket tells me she and her dad are about to be evicted. "Before he died—murdered—the nice man who let us stay here, free, never put anything in writing . . . I don't expect his son'll honor what his father told us."

Despite such a setback, Cricket is all smiles as she steps close to show me this small box she's painstakingly constructed that will hold Howard's memorial cards at his funeral service. "Like it?" she asks.

My "liking" this totem of death is a discordant thought. I've never known anyone, in such a matter-of-fact way, to discuss impending death. But I appraise the box. One side is wood, another brick, and the third stone. "This is really something," I say.

"Daddy's photo'll be attached to the fourth side. See . . ." She taps a gap separating two thin, neatly cut stone fragments. "In honor of his being a master mason, I used actual mortar."

## SEPTEMBER 19

Finishing *Lonesome Dove*, I'm about to start *Cold Mountain*. But Cricket wants to read something else. She holds up her draft eulogy and ticks off the twenty-eight professions or jobs Howard's held over the course of his eighty-four years: "Backhoe operator. Brick mason.

Pipe fitter." She looks up, proudly annotating, "Daddy's been certified a master of four different trades."

But Cricket misses one trade Howard had truly mastered. That of a drunk. "Put down *alcoholic*, Crick. I worked hard at that job." So hard he once swam home via a drainage canal—his booze-addled brain thinking the Lord had uncorked another epochal flood. "Daddy!" exclaimed Cricket at the door, after Howard's bacchanalia with his brick-laying buddies at the Dumfries Moose Lodge had left him drenched, inside and out. "How on earth did you get so wet?? It's hardly raining at all."

"The roads are all flooded, Crick. A disaster's befallen us. It's a deluge."

The next few months involve a deluge of transition-related details. Once evicted from the mobile home, Howard and Cricket relocate to the home of a relative. The move is difficult for all concerned.

Meanwhile, I'm trying to effect my own transition, by selling my minuscule Polish company to the $1 billion subsidiary of a Belgian conglomerate with $120 billion in assets. The principals get along great. The attorneys, not so much, which occasions numerous overseas trips and multiparty, multicity, multilingual conference calls. Many a day and night I long for a drink—ice-cold vodka shots, the tart and spritz of my reliable old friends, G & T, any number of the many deliciously flavorful, hammer-blow Belgian ales . . .

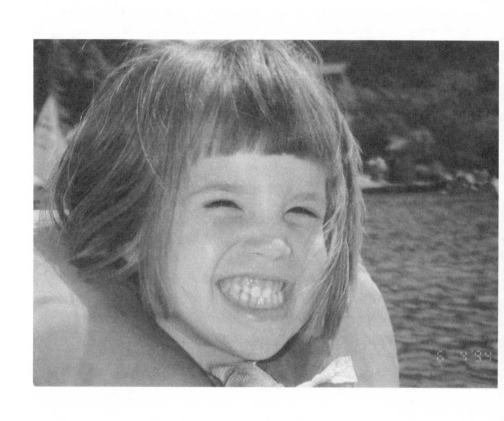

# LIVE DISCHARGE

Life is good. Normalcy has returned after fifteen months of intense, complex on-again/off-again negotiations. The sale of my company closed in Warsaw, on December 15. My eyes, hips, and parents are good. I'm catching up on my hikes with Ellen, as well as on my sleep and my reading.

## DECEMBER 29, 2011

It's a beautiful day, a harbinger for a great New Year. The Blue Ridge views are crisp, colorful. Fat squirrels are washing down acorns with water that's puddled atop our sunken well while crows caw and, every now and again, I'm treated to a honking squadron of Canada geese, flying southeasterly, in an imperfect but no less marvelous V-formation toward Old Rag Mountain. An Indian summer breeze slips through the open window, bringing with it a lovely aroma of burning logs and leaves, as our fluffy rescue dog, Alex, snores beside me on the bed, snuggling Ellen's pillow. My legs are propped up, and I'm reading the biography of a German theologian.

In walk Sarah and Ellen back from our daughter's twice-yearly appointment with her endocrinologist. (Whom she'd begun seeing following the detection of mild hypothyroidism during a routine sports physical in 2007, the summer before her junior year in high school. There were no symptoms.) Alex leaps down toward Ellen, who idles by the door as Sarah approaches the foot of the bed, twirling a long, auburn bang. My daughter pauses, close enough for me to notice that her lips are quivering. "Well . . ." she begins.

It takes a while for the facts to emerge. Sarah pauses every now and again to check the tears and find her voice. "The doctor saw something he didn't like on the sonogram. He couldn't feel it. But in checking my file, he could see it had grown since the last image. 'Hmm,' he says, and then makes this face. I knew it wasn't good. He says it could be cancer."

The word—*cancer*—freezes me, so much so that I don't even have the sense to hug Sarah, the thing she craves right now. My emotions are seized and crowded out by fleeting images of Rosalie's hair, kinked on account of her breast-cancer chemo, Gil's cancer-riddled kidney, Mara's nineteen-year-old son dying of brain cancer, Bob's metastasized prostate, and, of course, poor, bald Cricket, battling cancer throughout her tiny, rickety body. My entire hospice experience suddenly seems completely irrelevant, totally useless, and a colossal, selfish waste of time, like it's all been, rather than instructive, just the set-up for a cruel joke.

But then I see Dolly in my mind's eye, wagging her Neapolitan finger at me—and I get it. Following Alex's lead, I leap off the bed and embrace Sarah. "Tell me more."

Ellen takes over. "There's a twenty percent chance it's cancerous. But Dr. Tanen wants to do a biopsy." My wife touches Sarah's arm. "She was very brave. I don't know how she kept it together in Tanen's office and not cry."

"You kept me strong," says Sarah. "I kept my eyes on you. But my thoughts did start going crazy, as I imagine this thing growing in my neck. Whether or not it's cancer—whatever that means, exactly, other than something not good—just the fact that something is growing in my neck is really—literally, you know?—under my skin. I swear I think I'm gonna puke. But Mom sees I'm starting to lose it, and just her look calms me down. When Tanen steps out of the room for a moment, Mom says 'Let's not get ahead of ourselves. Doctors have to run lots and lots of tests, just to cover their butts, against lawsuits. I had to get a biopsy when pregnant with Matt. It turned out to be nothing.' This also calms me down. Some, anyway."

Meanwhile, I'm trying to keep it together, stay calm, and not exacerbate the anxiety. It's a real struggle.

The three of us go for a fine-needle biopsy. Two new doctors introduce themselves and explain what they're going to do. Sarah hates needles. Seeing that there are two needles—one to numb and a longer one to extirpate—makes her squirm, which she does in the sort of fancy, articulated, expensive-looking chair one sees in a dentist's office.

Sarah keeps it together as the first needle injects numbing meds into her neck. "We'll be back in a few minutes," the doctors say as they leave. Ellen and I look at Sarah, but she averts her eyes. Tearing up, she lifts her arm and dabs her eyes with her shirt sleeve.

After a few minutes, the doctors return and start preparing the second syringe, whose tip alone is longer than the length of the first syringe. Sarah looks away, grimacing, as the female member of this coed duo slowly inserts the gruesome-looking thin steel needle, pauses, then, with two fingers, pulls back on the device so as to retrieve a sample. Again the docs disappear.

After a while they return. The guy doc's trying not to stare off into the corner of the room as the woman, forthrightly panning her eyes back and forth amongst the three of us, says, "It is suspicious for papillary thyroid cancer. But we'd like to take another biopsy and send it off for a molecular test to try and get a more definitive answer."

We agree. Sarah endures two more needles, plus one more extraction.

Two weeks of waiting puts a damper on the New Year. However, the wait seems to have been worth it. The molecular test comes back negative for cancer.

But there's a hitch. As the test covers only twelve of the twenty potential genetic markers, many doctors never even use it, as such spotty coverage can give false hope.

We head back to Dr. Tanen's. The waiting room is packed, as would be expected, since he's one of the country's top endocrinologists. "Mark's great," says my friend and internist David Patterson, MD, who referred us to Tanen. "He doesn't miss much . . ." While Tanen couldn't feel the suspicious nodule during Sarah's physical exam, because it was so small, he was, first, seasoned enough to suggest the more discriminating

sonogram and, second, gifted enough to envision what was most likely going on, something many other docs surely would have missed.

Tanen's nowhere in sight, but a kindly lady ushers us into his compact
office, locating a third chair so we can all sit. His desktop includes one
of those digital frames that rotates photos every few seconds. To my left,
a squat glass-paned cabinet displays a collection of old patent medicine
bottles, antique advertising, and related memorabilia from his guild's
earlier days.

He enters, shakes our hands, and takes a seat. "So . . . want to hear
my opinion?"

Sarah's *yes* is atypically curt. Ellen and I nod.

"The tests are inconclusive," he says. "I still say twenty percent chance
it's cancer, though the newer test interprets things a bit differently."

"But," says Ellen, "some don't use the newer test because it has a
twenty percent chance of giving a false-negative result. Meaning the test
says it's all clear but it's not. Am I right?"

"You are," says Tanen, a smile almost breaking past the bulwark of his
all-business mien.

"So," I say, "Twenty percent yes, according to the older test, no per
the newer test—a test that yields erroneous results twenty percent of
the time?"

"You're right, too."

I follow up, "If it is cancer, do you have any idea what may have
caused it?"

"We really don't know. But I believe, in Sarah's case, as in most,
it's environmental. Maybe what the sonogram shows is benign, but I
doubt it. So there are three options. One, a total thyroidectomy, removing both glands. Two, a partial, removing just the gland where I
felt the nodule, then keep an eye on things. Three, sit tight and redo
the biopsy in three months."

Bob Zimmerman drifts into my head . . . whispering a key to unlock
some empathy. "What would you do, Dr. Tanen, were it your daughter?"

"The total. Even though all I got was a partial myself." He inserts two
fingers inside his shirt collar and tugs. "You should take some time to
think about it."

"Any downsides to doing a total?" Ellen asks.

Tanen shrugs, then cites boilerplate. "All surgery entails risk. But,
specifically, there are very few downsides—in Sarah's case, at least, as

her thyroid is hardly producing any of the hormone. Apart from that, the procedure would take, though not twice as long, a bit longer."

All the while Tanen's been talking, Sarah's been rapt, staring at him, studying him, trying to drink in every literal word, plus every hint suggested by his tone and body language.

"Doctor," I ask, "how much time do we have to think about which course to pursue?"

"Some."

"If she were to do the surgery," Ellen asks, "how involved is it and what's the post-op like? I'm thinking of her classes, at GW."

Tanen nods. Clearly he's heard this question before. "It all depends on what we find. If it has spread, Sarah would need to take radioactive iodine pills. She couldn't be around people for a few days, in classes, a dorm setting, et cetera."

I ask, "Is there any risk in waiting the four months or so until after the school year ends?"

"Not much. Thyroid cancer is not—typically—fast moving, and this mass, even if it is cancerous, is very small. It's more important to make the right decision and go about it right than to rush into it. If it's another type of cancer or if it were a big node or if I'd have found several or if there were any evidence that the cancer had started elsewhere, then it'd be a different story. Any other questions?" Clearly, he hopes the answer is no, at least not now, today, given his packed waiting room. Sarah, Ellen, and I exchange looks, rise, and leave.

On the ride back home, Sarah kicks things off by saying, "Option two seems pointless, and I never considered option three. Whether or not it's cancerous, having something—anything—growing in my neck just doesn't seem natural, and as for going back for check-ups and sonograms and biopsies, et cetera, I don't want that stress dogging me."

We discuss Tanen. We all think he really knows what he's doing, and his tendency, sometimes, to seem a bit abrupt is explained by his jam-packed waiting room.

Sarah says she's relieved that she'd girded herself for worse news. After the initial specter of cancer, she'd surfed the Internet and read how the survival rates for thyroid cancer are among the best of any type of cancer. So, she'd reasoned, there's a two-step process: First, it may not even be cancer, Tanen still giving it only a one-in-five chance that it is.

Second, even if it is cancer, the survival rates are really good, especially if the tumor is found early (as it has been) and the patient is young and in good health (as Sarah is).

Ellen's a bit more on edge, in part owing to the fact that her mother died of lung cancer after going back and forth, into and out of remission, not dying when doctors anticipated she would, then dying in a way and at a time that caught everyone off guard.

I'm not sure how I feel. But I do know that my side of the family hasn't had much experience with cancer. It's instead been bad hearts that have killed off many Lindners, some at a young age.

Once home, the three of us peel off to our respective coping mechanisms. After texting her best friend, Maria, and asking her to phone back, our athletic daughter (high school All-State in soccer and tennis, clutch on college varsity tennis, too) hits the gym. Ellen, from whom Sarah gets all her natural athleticism, would prefer going for a run or a swim, but duty calls her to the Internet. I text an old friend at Johns Hopkins Hospital, then, while waiting for him to respond, try to get a better handle on the numbers in an effort to quantify the situation.

The incidence of thyroid cancer has doubled over the past twenty years. (The suspected reasons include better testing and a host of environmental factors, including radiation, genetically modified and pesticide-"protected" foods, and the carcinogenic pressboards cranked out in China and used in millions of American homes in lieu of actual lumber, let alone plaster.) Circa 2012, nearly forty-five thousand new cases are reported in women, fifteen thousand in men. Each year, about two thousand people die of thyroid cancer. On average, the long-term survival rate for thyroid cancer is about 95 percent.

But I've never put much trust in "averages." In my experience, the "law of averages" is riddled with exceptions.

Nor do I find comfort in the B-school concepts of "Expected Value" or "hedging," which focus on the interplay of an outcome and its associated probability and maintain that, whenever one finds risk, so too will one find the potential for return. I can't hedge here. I see no potential return regarding Sarah's situation. A "mere" one-in-five chance of a terrible outcome is plenty bad.

Then my mind shifts from probability and statistics to chemistry and biology, to the issue of my genetic makeup and medical history—of which, obviously and unfortunately, Sarah is heir. Several doctors have told me, "Eric, you deserve your own chapter in a medical textbook, entitled 'Statistical Deviation.'" My corneas are massive, my hip sockets tiny, the arches of my feet freakishly high, and, as several of my high school classmates loved to note, my dense, pointy, elongated head does indeed resemble an anvil. In other words, when it comes to me, my organs, my hormones, my DNA—in other words, the primary arbiters of Sarah's condition—what's average, typical, expected, and "normal" goes right out the window.

Ellen's historical perspective adds to our augury. She's been especially cursed by the laws of probability and statistics. For instance, it was astronomically improbable that once three of his four engines had given out in September 1963 her pilot father, while flying five hundred miles from land (Ireland), not much closer to the nearest vessel, buffeted by thirty-five-knot winds and fifteen-foot, near-freezing waves, would be able to ditch his passenger plane at 2:30 A.M. in the North Atlantic. But Captain John Murray did, miraculously saving forty-eight lives, getting himself the biggest parade in the history of Oyster Bay, Long Island, and landing his cut and bandaged face in the *Saturday Evening Post*, whose cover story was "Miracle Pilot Ditches at Sea!" Statistically speaking, it was only slightly less probable that her expert swimmer and heroic dad would then drown three years later while scuba diving off Wake Island. Such an early trauma had taught Ellen . . . whenever the seas start white capping and the wind starts picking up . . . to make ready. So she hits the Internet, reviewing the latest clinical studies . . . so, when we confer with Sarah's doctors, we'll do so, in the words of Bill Gates, "at a high bandwidth, in real time." At a minimum, her research tells her that we need to get a second opinion.

Prior to this "mass, suspicious of cancer," things with Sarah had been going great. She loves George Washington, the university to which she'd transferred as a second-semester sophomore ten months prior to her diagnosis. Though beginning as an American studies major, she had—co-incidentally—fallen in love with her health and wellness courses, and so she'd added this as a minor. Her enviable internships included Washington Speakers' Bureau, where Colin Powell and other leaders graciously offered her tips, and a fascinating, community-service oriented healthcare start-up that, like Google, Apple, and so many bright ideas, two guys were trying to launch from their basement. Also, after experiencing the full spectrum of college-age male morons, she'd finally met someone she felt she could be herself with, who—having served several tours in war zones—helped her put her battle into perspective.

While waiting for my Hopkins friend to respond to my text, my eyes drift around my home office, which used to be Matt's bedroom before he'd left for California. On the wall, above the mothballed fireplace, is artwork pertaining to each of my kids: the painted logo of Matt's first firehouse, Company 11, based in Orlean, Virginia, and a pen-and-ink drawing of a groundhog, which Sarah did earlier in 2011, a few weeks after our first meeting with Tanen.

I've seen lots of pen-and-inks by Rembrandt and other masters. Brueghel (the Younger) is my favorite. But I'd not trade a single one for any of Sarah's masterpieces, most especially not the one of this fat pest. When groundhogs overran (over-waddled) our home, burrowing under our foundation, into our HVAC system, a week before I was to head off to Europe, after more humane methods failed (such as traps set by a local game warden), I bought my first rifle and set about trying to rid our property of them. After hours of lying in wait, from our second floor, I had little to show for it: one dead, one winged, dozens unharmed. When I returned from Europe, Sarah had a present for me tacked to the front door: her masterpiece. Somehow, she'd managed to make her groundhog look both fierce and silly. Above the varmint's head is a simple taunt: "Welcome Back."

This isn't to say that our father-daughter relationship has been frictionless. Well into her toddlehood she wanted nothing at all to do with me—clinging to her mother, looking at me as if I were some strange, horrible monster. Since then, we've had run-ins over friends, curfews, priorities. She's lashed out at me, her mom, her brother.

But come the time of her ambivalent diagnosis, Sarah and I have a very unambivalent relationship. Akin to Dolly's modus operandi, Sarah often communicates in coded tones and body language that often confuse her mother and—always—irritate the hell out of her older brother. Sarah employs myriad different smiles, eye rolls, and quips, such as, "I'm in a meeting!" which she'll lob out as we pass someone yakking away on their cell phone for all the world to hear, taking themselves entirely too seriously.

My cell phone rings. It's Roger Blumenthal. "What's up, E?"

Though "only" one of the world's top heart doctors, probably the planet's premier preventive cardiologist, Roger is legendary not only for the range of his medical expertise but also for his willingness to drop anything to help a friend. While his friends include the high and mighty, Roger and I are best friends; what's more, he's Sarah's godfather. "Thanks for calling back, R, and so quickly."

"'Course, 'course. What's going on?"

Wanting to be respectful of his time, I'm succinct, clinical. I tell him I called to see if he might be able to recommend a top-notch second opinion to help us get a better grasp of Sarah's situation, which I then summarize.

Once I'm done, and he's offered condolences, he asks some follow-up questions. Like so many who are tops in their field (whatever the field), Roger is amazingly humble. He exudes the single-mindedness and presence that I aspire to but rarely attain when visiting hospice patients. Though he seems to pack seventy-two hours of work into every twenty-four hours, Roger never talks fast, like everyone did at law school, and he never makes one feel like he's rushed, like his time is more valuable than yours (like many doctors do).

As I'd hoped, it turns out that Roger doesn't just know a fair bit about thyroid cancer or know of a good second opinion, he knows the world's leading researcher in the field, who, like so many experts, is also based at Hopkins. "E, Dr. Ball sometimes collaborates with Wendy." (Wendy Post, MD, is Roger's cardiologist wife.)

"Incredible, R! I knew you'd come through! You always do!"

## FEBRUARY 10

Another friend comes through, as well: Cricket. During a visit, when she hears of Sarah's potential cancer, she says, "I know Sarah's worried, so let's go shooting."

"What? You're serious?"

"I am."

"I don't know, Cricket. Sarah's pretty emotional right now."

"I'm sure she is. That exactly why it'd be great for her to shoot the crap out of something."

"What??" Sarah exclaims, when, later in the day, I pass along Cricket's suggestion.

"It's more than that," I say. "She's been battling cancer for a long time. I think she has more in mind than sharing a few tips on marksmanship."

"But I've never even met her. You ever shoot with her, Dad?"

"No. But Matt has. You might ask him about it. I say, her asking you is a real honor."

"What's she like?"

"She's crazy. And ornery."

"Crazy? You want me to go shooting . . . with someone who's crazy . . . and ornery??"

"Both in a good way. Crazy like your favorite singer, Miranda Lambert. Gunpowder-and-lead ornery. I don't think you'll be disappointed. She thinks it'll help you take your mind off . . ."

"Sure, then. I'm game. Why not?"


## FEBRUARY 13

Sarah, Cricket, and I agree to rendezvous in the Warrenton Sheetz parking lot, just off Route 29. Sarah follows me in her car, as I plan to head over to visit Howard. Cricket's already there when we arrive. Sarah hops into Cricket's rust-riddled Chrysler minivan (that's at least as old as Sarah) and waves to me as they head south, while I head north.

What Sarah notices first is how Cricket's wearing really big, baggy clothes, "I'm guessing to hide how her body looks. She's smoking constantly but asks, once, if it's okay, if I mind, because she could put it out. Even though I do mind, especially in the car, I'm not going to tell a woman dying to stop doing one action that allows her some pleasure/joy."

At Clark Brothers, Cricket's a celebrity: parts Annie Oakley, parts Charlton Heston, 100 percent break-the-mold unique. Clark Brothers is where she bought her monster revolver, and it's where everyone knows her name. Her version of Cheers. Guys yell, "Hey, Cricket!" and others ask about her father . . . She waves, saying how much Howard misses seeing everybody.

The gun range is behind the shop, and Cricket marches onto the covered platform like her name is Clark, not Cooper. She ignores all the guys, who take a break from shooting to observe and elbow each other regarding this Odd Couple: the only representatives of the feminine gender;

an athletic 5'9", the smiling Sarah towers over the sullen Cricket, who ignores all the posted signs, including the one that says "ALL ammo must be purchased in the shop—NO EXCEPTIONS!" Cricket shakes her box of ammo and gives Sarah a look. "Bought this at Wal-Mart."

Her two guns she lays on the wooden table at the end of the range: a .380 Sig Sauer automatic and a Dan Wesson .44 mag long barrel. "She tells me to go ahead and pick them up, look them over, get comfortable with them." The .44 is huge and heavy, weighing in at five pounds. Cricket loads both guns, explains some safety tips, how to stand, aim, etc. "Then she starts shooting, as if it were just a normal part of her day. She's good! I stand back watching her go a few rounds, still quite nervous to be about to hold a gun, and with all the gunshots going off around me."

"You're up," says Cricket, as she reloads the pistol, then hands it over.

Sarah shakes her head and gathers her long, thick hair in a band. Hair so long and thick that, though he envies her endowment, Sarah's stylist charges her extra because it takes him so much longer to cut. Such an endowment that one of my favorite family pictures is of Baby Sarah, struggling to hold her head up in the maternity ward nursery under the weight of her black mop, which, after her first baby bath and shampoo, was so abnormally full that all the nurses crammed around the viewing window to observe the freakish feline mane. Not only does Sarah tower over Cricket but also she's got forty pounds more muscle, too, which powers her pro caliber, one hundred mph tennis serve. Yet Sarah almost drops the five-pound gun, prompting a cackle. "You'll get used to it," says Cricket.

"Cricket doesn't rush me . . . tells me to wait until I'm ready . . . to relax. 'Shoot on Sarah time.' She laughs at me for how timid I'm being and re-minds me not to turn the gun toward anyone after shooting. My first shot hits the target. She raises her eyebrows, quite surprised at my being able to hit the target on my first try. As I continue shooting I begin to feel more comfortable. The rest of the range has gotten silent. All the guys eyeing us . . . checking out the chicks with the cannon . . . blowing the target to smithereens. Cricket and I give each other a look, and laugh."

In between shooting, laughing, loading, and reloading, Cricket talks to Sarah about her dad. Not the current—bad, sad—stuff. Just the good stuff. How Howard used to take "Crick" hunting when she was really young and how much she loved it.

Cricket delves into a very dark corner of hunting, too, telling Sarah, "The best way to make sure no one messes with you is to carry a gun and to make sure everyone knows it."

Sarah explains how the last thing her inner-city college wants are students with guns. "Predators know this," Cricket says. She urges Sarah to get a gun permit, at the very least, if and when she starts living on her own. "Women got to protect themselves and their families."

Sarah invites Cricket to lunch. It's on their way that Cricket broaches the subject of cancer. She starts off generally, talking about how important it is not to let cancer—or the prospect of it—rule one's life, how it's really important to get second opinions, to really question doctors and really push them. Then she asks about the specifics of Sarah's situation. "As we're passing the hospital, I say how we're still in the 'gray' area of not knowing, how my parents are worried but we're all staying positive." Cricket gets into the particulars of thyroid cancer, reassuring Sarah that thyroid is the best cancer to have since it's the slowest growing. "If you're going to have cancer, thyroid's the one you want." Cricket also confirms what the doctors have said: that the cure rate is especially high if the cancer is discovered early in your life and you're healthy.

They stop at an Italian place beside Route 29, in the heart of Warrenton, where Cricket orders a panino, Sarah a slice. As Cricket eats her big sandwich and talks of bull's-eyes as a proxy for living life to the fullest . . . a sublime comprehension begins to dawn on Sarah. "I feel blessed, that I should be grateful. Seeing her . . . a woman dying of all forms of cancer . . . waking up each day . . . marching forward . . . seemingly fearless . . . makes me think, What the hell am I complaining for?" Sarah's not sure if it's "a test from above, or what," but she is sure, from that moment on, that "I'll get through this, and I'll be stronger because of it."

Sarah doesn't eat much of her cheese pizza. Cricket wolfs half of her cheese-and-pepperoni behemoth and gets the rest wrapped to go. Sarah offers to pay. "It was such a small thing . . . but she accepted with so much more gratitude than most people, when accepting a free meal. Afterward, once I'd dropped her off and she'd headed home, I felt lighter . . . as if some of the worry had been . . . shot away."

Fifteen minutes later, at home, my wife and I sitting at the kitchen table, talking, fretting, we hear Sarah come in through the front door. Ellen and I glance at each other, apprehensively. Sarah enters the kitchen—

beaming. She holds up her target, shot to hell. "Oh . . . my . . . God! I've never had so much fun in my life! I can't wait to go again!" As she starts removing her scarf, a spent shell pops out, clanking to the kitchen floor.

"You just be sure," I say, "to do that the next time you're at some bar and a guy who doesn't interest you gets a little too close."

Cancer now the furthest thing from her mind, Sarah bursts out laughing and buckles over. My wife and I have never seen her laugh so hard. We join her.

## FEBRUARY 17

Though such a humble guy, he'd never say so, but Dr. Douglas Ball is probably the world's top thyroid researcher. When he enters the cramped room at John Hopkins, Sarah, Ellen, and I immediately sense that he's 180 degrees from Dr. Tanen. Poor Tanen always seems so rushed, like he has, if he's lucky, two minutes per patient, whereas Ball looks totally relaxed as he collapses into a rolling chair, leaning back as it skits across the floor, as if to say, "Take as much time as you need. I've got all time in the world."

But after a brief introduction what he actually says is, "I had my team review the original biopsies, and our assessment is a bit different. We don't rate it as 'suspicious for cancer.' We rate it 'atypical, of uncertain significance.'"

We're not sure what to make of these semantics. We'd come to Ball in the hope of finding greater clarity, amid, for one thing, two competing 20 percent probabilities. Now he adds yet another layer of opaqueness.

On the other hand, *uncertain* seems a heck of a lot better than *suspicious of cancer*. But we're not sure it changes anything material. We're still inclined to proceed with a total thyroidectomy, based on Tanen's recommendation, which includes the facts that the removal of Sarah's thyroid would eliminate any potential "cancer host" and, as her thyroid is pretty much not functioning at all now (the hormones provided by pills), it seems to make sense to remove the defunct organ, akin to an appendectomy. So, as we still need a surgeon, we file Ball's new diagnostic twist away as we proceed to our next Hopkins appointment with Dr. Sara Pai. Ball sends us on our way with some friendly advice: "Don't let how young she looks fool you. Sara is very experienced and very, very good."

I'm glad we'd been warned, because had she not been wearing a white coat, with her name and *MD* embroidered on it, I would have thought Dr. Pai had taken a wrong turn on the way to the nearest high school. Beyond her youthful look, the first thing that catches my eye is her shoe size. Her feet are tiny. She must either love—or hate—shopping.

Sarah notices something much more germane: right off the bat, Dr. Pai looks her in the eye and smiles. This simple, human connection puts Sarah at ease, visibly.

I'm put at ease by a different trait: Dr. Pai's habit, like Elmer's, of finding humor, despite the seriousness of the situation. She starts with the coincidence in first names—her not having an H on the end of hers strikes her as hilarious. However, in between the bouts of laughter that rattle her minute body, one gets the clear impression that here sits a lady who's not about to rattle when things get tough. This tiny doctor with the titanic skill set is just the sort you want in your corner if things get dicey.

However, Dr. Pai adds yet another layer to our confusion, telling us that just as Ball didn't fully concur with Tanen, she doesn't fully concur with Ball, either. The gist of Pai's assessment is that she's not so sure surgery is warranted. "I know the perception is that surgeons are supposed to be the ones always wanting to operate, but that's not me." Her focus, she explains, is the total picture, a holistic outcome, and from what she's seen she's not convinced that calls for a thyroidectomy, partial or whole. Dr. Pai is inclined to wait and see whether additional tests, such as a repeat biopsy, should be done before surgery, and she wants to talk things over more with Drs. Ball and Tanen.

Ellen, Sarah, and I exchange looks, not sure what to say. But, as we figure we're here, with this ace, super-busy surgeon, whom Tanen and Ball both recommended, we might as well get a little smarter on the surgical side of things, in the event we elect to go the operation route. "Can we still ask a few questions?" Ellen begins.

"Sure!" says Dr. Pai, seemingly delighted by the notion.

"I understand that one of the biggest risks," says Ellen, "is accidentally nicking the vocal cords when removing the thyroid. Is that right? Have you ever had any problems?"

Dr. Pai's mien is now all business. "Yes, it can be a tricky procedure. But as for me, I've been very fortunate. I've never damaged the vocal cords."

I jump in. "How many times, if I might ask, have you performed this sort of surgery?"

Dr. Pai turns to me, smiles, and nods. "Hundreds."

Ellen, Sarah, and I exchange more looks: of relief and an appreciation for the deft way Dr. Pai is able to express her self-confidence but in such a humble way.

Ellen asks how long the procedure normally takes. Dr. Pai caveats her answer but says that in Sarah's case it would probably take between one and a half and two hours. "Most of the time would involve taking care to find and protect the vocal cord nerves so they don't get damaged."

Ellen asks about the recovery, including the time needed, and what creams to use to ensure the neck scar heals flush with the skin with a minimum of discoloration. When Dr. Pai says the recovery period would be two weeks, Ellen asks, "Would it be possible after the recovery period that we three go to Hawaii for an extended vacation? I'd like Sarah to have something really fun to look forward to after surgery."

"Hawaii!" exclaims Dr. Pai, triggering another bout of giggling. "That is awesome!" She tells us how having grown up in California she often visits Hawaii and hopes to retire there. She assures us there would be "no problem whatsoever" with Sarah visiting, even for six weeks. But Dr. Pai does tell Sarah she'd have to be sure to cover the neck area not only with a total sunblock but also with a fabric. "The Hawaiian sun is very hot, being so near the equator and I don't want your scar to get discolored. I wish I was going with you."

"One more thing, Doctor?" I say, prodded by Ellen's thorough research.

"Call me Sara. Yes?"

"If we do go forward with the operation, could we ask that it only be you who does the actual procedure? It's just that . . ."

Dr. Pai nods. "We are a teaching hospital, and I will have some students and residents by my side. I am in the operating room the entire time from when Sarah goes to sleep to when she wakes up from anesthesia. I will handle all of the tricky areas around the vocal cord nerves."

## MARCH 18

It's a busy Sunday. By this time, we've met with seven different doctors as well as countless nurses and technicians. These meetings have been supplemented by phone calls, e-mails, and Internet searches. We need to make a decision.

Actually, we need to make a series of decisions. One big thing has to do with locking down Dr. Pai. She's in such high demand, we could only get on her wait list. If we're going the surgical route, it's time to commit. Though we would still not know the actual date of surgery until a few days in advance (which adds to our anxiety), if we want to remain on the wait list we need to let her know, which is only common courtesy. If, on the other hand, we've decided not to do the surgery or wish to wait a little longer, say, do it over the Christmas break in 2012, again, we need to let her know. There are a lot of people with serious problems that Dr. Pai can help, so it's time for us to put an end to our paralysis of analysis.

Not just yet, however. We have a final consult with Dr. Tanen, confer with Drs. Patterson and Blumenthal, and surf the Internet a few final times, just for good measure, to see if we might have missed something or, in the intervening weeks, some new data, procedures, or other relevant information has arisen that should be thrown into the hopper. Sarah, Ellen, and I share a final round of ideas, thoughts, hopes, and fears.

We continue to involve Matt. Though at times they squabble (their screams across the house sometimes bloodcurdling), Matt and Sarah are much closer than I was with my sister at a similar age. (The fault being mine, entirely.) Matt can be gruff, but in this instance he's sensitive, rightly striking an encouraging note. He reminds of us of a girl we all know, also in college, who a few years back had a different type of cancer. It also came out of the blue. It was very frightening for our friends, likewise the parents of a son and daughter. "She's totally okay now," Matt reminds us.

While I've told my parents what's going on, I've not told my siblings. Nor have I told any friends, apart from Roger. Sarah, Ellen, and I felt a semi-strict policy of "need to know" made the most sense, at least until we got a better handle on things.

Though I'm honestly not sure how good a handle I've got on things, during one of my regular Sunday visits I decide to inform Gordon's widow. Having met Sarah, Dorothy is always inquiring into her well-being. Since the appearance of Sarah's possible cancer, each time I've dissembled I've felt guilty.

I feel especially guilty here, now, as I open up about Sarah's situation. Dorothy looks stoic. I infer a tinge of surprise but not a whiff of anger or even displeasure. I sense she's a bit taken aback, seeing how we've been friends now for more than two years, delving into a number of delicate, sensitive areas, including others we know who've fought cancer; some successfully, some not. "We've not told hardly anyone," I say. "Everyone has issues they're dealing with. We've not wanted to burden anyone."

"I understand." She proceeds to unburden me, telling me how her sister had a thyroidectomy, as have several other friends and loved ones. Though I'm somewhat afraid to inquire about the results, I do. "Why, they all just fine!" Dorothy has not a single problem to report, even though some of the thyroid cancers she cites weren't discovered until the women were twice Sarah's age and the patients weren't anywhere near as fit as Sarah. "You'd never know they had cancer. Live life just the same, can't hardly see no scar."

That evening, Sarah commits to surgery. The prospect of her dying still seems remote, but it's as real and certain as the image on the sonogram. It's as real and certain as Gordon Ford and all my other hospice patients dying, without a single live discharge. It's as real and certain as Ellen's dad defying astronomical odds to live; only, in a commonplace cosmic coda, to drown. It's as real as Heisenberg's uncertainty principle.

Though we've committed to surgery, we've yet to decide whether to remove just one thyroid gland or both. Three outstanding doctors all come down slightly differently regarding what we should do. After one final, lengthy, late-night telephone consult with a gracious and empathetic Dr. Ball, we decide to do the total thyroidectomy.


## MAY 17

As Sarah can't eat or drink past midnight (water included) and must be at the hospital by 5:30 A.M. on the 18th, for a scheduled 7:30 A.M. surgery, we decide to overnight in Baltimore rather than awaken at 2:30 A.M. and drive from our Warrenton home. It also allows us to grab dinner at one of Little Italy's terrific, authentic family owned restaurants.

Whenever in Charm City it's our standing policy to spend time with
Roger Blumenthal; his delightful mother, Anita; his lovely, super-bright
fellow Hopkins doc–wife, Wendy; and their kinetic, iconoclastic son,
Ross, who, though he now vastly prefers lacrosse and golf, seems teed
up for something other than sports, given his DNA. But this go 'round
none of us feels up to "entertaining." At dinner, Sarah gets her regular:
pasta with chicken and marinara. Ellen gets salmon. I opt for veal. We
talk about a number of things but not the surgery. Our table is the quiet-
est in the place, by far.

The morning of surgery, Sarah starts off calm. There's little talking during our short drive to Johns Hopkins Hospital. Arriving on the sixth floor
of Weinberg at 5:17 A.M., we join a handful of other nervous-looking
people at intake and are warmly greeted by a blue-smocked woman who
tells us what we can expect, including regular updates. Sarah is escorted
off to get prepped for surgery while Ellen and I are ushered into a large,
well-appointed waiting lounge, where, like clusters of other families
huddled about, we alternate between ignoring altogether and staring
blankly at one of several TVs suspended from the ceiling.

At 7:20, we're invited back into the pre-op waiting area. Sarah is no
longer calm, but she's putting on a brave face. "I feel cold, hungry,
and afraid but also lucky and loved." Loved on account of the looks
she's receiving from strangers that say, *I'm not sure why you're here,
sweetie, but we're sorry, and we're sure rooting for you*, and the af-
fectionate questions she gets from the nurses, such as, "You're not
pregnant now, sweetie, are you?" Sarah feels lucky because she's much
better off than many around her, such as "this small girl, maybe eight
years old, in a wheelchair. Her eyes are red and tired looking; she's
struggling to keep them open. Her parents are staring at the floor,
looking really sad. I can't imagine worse pain for a parent, seeing your
young child expecting death or the very real possibility of dying. This
makes me feel awful but also lucky. I almost break down. I try not to
stare at them or catch their eyes. I really want to hug them." Sarah's
afraid for two reasons. First, "because most around me are either
really young or really old. At twenty-one, I seem so out of place."
Second, whether young or old, most around her seem in really bad
shape, more like the little girl than like Sarah, underscoring the seri-

ous nature of happy Dr. Pai's trade, which required Sarah to sign a set of waivers acknowledging and agreeing that anything could go wrong, "up to and including death." Sarah is hungry because the pasta's been fully digested and the stomach needs to be empty so the anesthesia can be dosed correctly. Finally, she's cold because the thermometer is set low to inhibit the spread of bacteria.

But the anesthesiologist relaxes Sarah, in more ways than one. "This'll feel like you've had a few margaritas, is all. Then you'll be in dreamland. Then you'll wake up."

"Hold up," Sarah says. "Can I use the bathroom, first?"

"Sure. Over there." He points.

Grabbing and pinching the back of her flimsy gown, she pads her way to the bathroom, located just before the OR doors. Unbeknownst to Ellen and me, while going about her business, Sarah is interrupted by a male patient, in his forties, who walks in on her (the lock was broken). "My jaw just dropped in embarrassment." As she exits the bathroom, she sees the guy rush toward his bed and yank the curtain shut, apparently every bit as embarrassed as she. When she returns to Ellen and me, huddled beside her bed, whispering anxiously, Sarah exclaims, "Good news!"

"How so?" says Ellen.

Sarah points at the still-rustling curtain. "See that guy who just went in behind there?"

Ellen and I shrug, and shake our heads.

"Well he walked right in on me in the bathroom, as I was peeing."

"Oh, no!" Ellen exclaims.

"But yes, *Maja*! You know how Dad always says if something starts out bad it's going to end up good. So it's a sign." Sarah climbs back onto her gurney bed. Ellen hugs her, kisses her on the forehead, and says, "It'll all be over soon, and it's going to be alright." I hug her, kiss her, and say, "Listen to your mom." Sarah is wheeled into the OR, and we head back out into the waiting area.

Ninety minutes later, Ellen and I are fidgeting. We'd been told we'd get regular updates, but we've received none, even though, according to Dr. Pai, the operation might only take ninety minutes. Everyone around us seems to be getting their updates—by the looks of it some good, some not so good.

Near the two-hour mark, a woman approaches us and relays a brief boilerplate update, which, so far as I can tell, allows us to infer only that our daughter is still alive and still being operated on. Thereafter, every twenty minutes or so, I make trips to the main desk to inquire what the heck is going on, but all I'm told is either "There's nothing new to report" or "All we know is that your daughter is still in the OR." Finally, at the four-hour mark, a woman walks up to us, makes sure we are attentive, and says, "The surgery is over, and your daughter is in recovery."

"How'd it go?" says Ellen. "When can we see Sarah?"

"Your doctor will be out to see you shortly."

A few minutes later, Dr. Pai is rushing toward us—the picture of her big smile worth more than a thousand words. She sits beside us. She looks exhausted. "It went great. Just much longer than expected. We never know what we'll encounter until we actually get inside."

"What did you encounter?" Ellen asks.

"Some inflammation and scarring due to Sarah's chronic lymphocytic thyroiditis. There was just one small, really hard node in her thyroid gland. Really hard. But it was a big success."

"No cancer, then?" I ask.

"Not in any of the lymph nodes I sampled to evaluate for cancer spread. But we'll have to wait for the final pathology of the thyroid gland itself. That could take up to ten days."

More waiting, more puzzlement. Ellen and I glance at one another. Silently we exchange the same thought: How come they know instantly about the lymph nodes but must wait ten days to find out about the thyroid glands? But we let it slide for the time being, because, first, we don't want anything holding us up from seeing Sarah and, second, we know the surgery's extended duration has been hard on Dr. Pai, who's struggling to be present with us, although we can tell she's a bit antsy, probably to get some lunch, before heading off to her next surgery—hours behind schedule.

"We don't want to keep you," I say. "We . . ." I look at Ellen, hoping she concurs with me that it's best to defer more questions so as to not delay seeing Sarah. Ellen concurs. "You must be tired," I continue. "And hungry! Thank you so much, Dr. Pai."

"Yes," says Ellen. "Thank you very much. Can we see Sarah now?"

"Sure." Dr. Pai nods at the aide who'd informed us the surgery was over. Ellen and I take turns shaking Dr. Pai's hand, and then she dashes off while the aide escorts us from the waiting room into the recovery suite.

While we've been outside, Sarah's anesthesia has worn off—too fast. She's heard nothing about the results of her surgery. She can't talk. But she can cry, and her thoughts can race. What have they found? Was it cancer? How much? Where? How fast was it growing? Is it growing just in my neck or other places, too?? What if they only think they got it all but really missed some?? Even if they got it all, what about my voice? The Internet has all these horror stories! What about Maria's friend who had to undergo chemo and radiation? Will all my hair fall out?? And what's the deal with all the pain!? Dr. Pai told me there wouldn't be much pain, but there's tons!

"Then you and Mom walk in. At first, it's worse, because I see the worried look on your faces, and it just feeds back and doubles up on my own worries and fears—so I cry harder.

"Mom rushes beside me, leans down, presses her head against mine, and strokes my hair. I think this must have triggered a bucket of tears, because I remember just letting it all hang out."

"Poor baby," Ellen says. Then almost as an afterthought, she adds, "When did they last give you your pain medication?"

Sarah shakes her head.

"What do you mean?" I say, after hugging her and kissing her. "You've not had any recently?"

With her neck bandaged, Sarah has the presence of mind not to shake her head forcefully. But her movement is perceptible enough; she squeezes my hand, staring into my eyes as tears dribble down her cheeks. Ellen daubs them while I say, "What are you saying? Are you saying since waking from the anesthesia they've not given you any-thing?!" Another hand squeeze and more tears.

I turn to Ellen just as she turns to me. I kiss Sarah on the forehead then head off.

After a few moments, I'm back with a nurse. She seems pleasant enough, but her comment is unacceptable: "Dr. Pai doesn't ordinarily like to give narcotics following thyroid surgery."

"This isn't an ordinary situation," I say, trying not to lose my temper. "Ordinarily, the procedure takes one and a half, maybe two hours. Our daughter, Sarah, here—look at her, please, will you?? She was in there for . . . four hours. Now I understand the anesthesia may have been supplemented to account for the longer duration, but, still, the fact remains, Dr. Pai said Sarah would not—should not—be experiencing much—if any—pain . . . post-op. Yet here she is, as you can plainly see . . . experiencing pain. Quite a lot of pain."

"I'll check with the doctor," says the nurse.

"Please," I say. "Sarah here has a high tolerance for pain, and I myself have had nearly twenty operations, many here at Hopkins. And this is not right. I know this is not right."

The nurse returns, quickly. Before long, Sarah's hooked up to an IV, and the painkiller starts doing its thing.

The next morning, as Ellen and I enter her hospital room, Sarah looks pale, haggard, and, unusually, makes little effort to smile. Ellen and I stroke her hair, kiss her, hold her hand, and praise her courage, maturity, and stoicism. "Dr. Pai said it went great," says Ellen. "Just longer than expected. How'd you sleep?"

Sarah starts crying but then holds up her iPod, the music on which is audible. "Enya," I say. "Relaxing," she whispers, her first post-op words to us. "A little."

A nurse arrives, says hello, and starts fiddling with a velcro strap near Sarah's ankle. It's noisy, annoying, and disruptive.

"Compression?" I ask.

"Yes," says the nurse, "to prevent blood clots."

I look to Sarah, who rolls her eyes. "How often?" I ask.

"Every few hours," says the nurse.

"You did it every few hours, during the night, too?"

"Yes."

Ellen looks my way, prompting me to ask, "Is this really necessary?"

"Yes, until Sarah can walk around, to get the blood flowing on her own."

"Walk around for how long?" I ask.

"Ten minutes," says the nurse, "every two hours."

I look to Ellen, who nods.

I look to Sarah. "Let's roll," she whispers, hoarsely, throwing off the cover.

The following day, once back home in Virginia, the recovery regresses. Sarah's bandage is gone, but her throat is still red and raw-looking. The OxyContin controls the neck pain but at the cost of a splitting headache that makes Sarah want to cry and vomit; so both her head and neck are throbbing. She's whispering a bit more, but just the bare essentials, when absolutely necessary. "It's the worst I feel, through the whole thing. I'm on the couch, downstairs, crying because of the pain, the nausea, the dizziness, feeling so tired—but not being able to sleep. Mom gets me a cold towel and tries to calm me down, relax me. She starts massaging my feet. I can feel her love without her saying a word.

"Then you come in. I can tell you feel horrible for me. You look really concerned. You urge me to try to get down some pain medicine and go upstairs to sleep. I nod, so Mom gets me some meds; then you both help me up into a sitting position, off the couch. Then you walk me upstairs."

A few days later, things are much improved. The bandage is off, and though the neck still looks pretty bad, the pain is much better. Sarah is off the OxyContin completely, only taking Tylenol occasionally. On the other hand, she's still not getting much sleep or eating much, the latter both because of some lingering nausea and because it hurts to swallow. Given the lack of sleep and calories, Sarah looks wan. While she's in her room, asleep (or at least resting), listening to Enya, Ellen and I are upstairs, across the hall from one another, tending to e-mails, many from friends and family inquiring how Sarah's doing and how we're doing.

But all the while we're tap-tapping away, Ellen and I are wondering, *When will Dr. Pai call to share the biopsy results?* As Sarah is twenty-one, she has the right to be informed first. But she'd okayed Dr. Pai talking with us first.

We're not on edge, however. Dr. Pai's report was so positive. Sarah is finally getting some rest, eating some food. As life is returning to normal, Ellen and I are experiencing a sense of relief that's been absent for not just weeks but months.

Dr. Pai calls Ellen. Seeing my wife wave at me, I rush over and sit beside her. Ellen hits the speakerphone button and then says, "Eric just got here. We're on speakerphone."

"Hi, Dr. Pai," I say.

"Hi," she responds, her voice as chipper as ever. "How's Sarah doing?"

"Much better," says Ellen. "But it was a rough first few days."

"I'm really sorry about the post-op pain," says the doctor. "Well, we've got the pathology results back, from the thyroid . . ."

Ellen and I don't look at each other, but we squeeze hands.

"It was cancerous after all."

Now my wife and I look at each other. Ellen's head droops, as her hand goes to her mouth. "It was?" I say.

"Yes," says Dr. Pai.

Ellen and I don't know what to say. But some disconcerting thoughts begin to reemerge. Neither of us gave it much thought—that the rock-like mass Dr. Pai had removed from Sarah's neck would indeed prove to be cancerous. Such a prospect just receded into the background, what with the negative results from the surrounding lymph nodes and the ever-smiling Dr. Pai's post-op happy talk.

Dr. Pai puts our minds at ease, or tries to. "But there's no sign, at all, that the cancer had spread beyond the thyroid gland based on the lymph nodes that were removed and were all negative for having cancer. All of the cancer was removed; there was no sign of cancer in the margins around the gland or evidence of cancer going into the bloodstream within the thyroid gland. This means Sarah will not need to take radioactive iodine pills or undergo any other treatment. Sarah will live just as long, enjoying the same quality of life, as if she'd never had cancer. The fact that we caught it so soon made the difference. It may have saved Sarah's life."

But there's no "may" about it. Not in my book, anyway. Nor is there any *we*, either, no slight implied as regards Dr. Pai's remarkable surgical skills, Tanen's diagnostic talent, etc. It's really very simple: in my book, Ellen saved Sarah's life. I look over at my wife, bite my lip, and begin to blubber, so thankful at her having been so vigilant over the past six years . . . While I've been focused on investing in Polish parking lots, she's been investing in something that really matters to me. I feel like an idiot and a fool—serendipitously snatched from a nightmare of my own making.

Ellen says, "How about calcium pills?"

"No," says Dr. Pai. "No need to take any calcium supplements, either. Just checkups every six months and ultrasounds at least for a couple years."

Once we say our final thanks to Dr. Pai and hang up, Ellen and I remain seated. We both feel numb. We know we should—once again—feel blessed, given Dr. Pai's prognosis and all, but the totally unexpected reintroduction of the word *cancer*—after five long months, the first actual confirmation of any malignancy—embeds in our relief an irreducible node of anxiety.

Our immediate concern, now, is tactical: when, how, and what to tell Sarah, which of the two of us should do the talking, and so on. As we sit, whispering conspiratorially . . . I think back on how and when Rosalie's cancer was first confirmed, Gil Booker's, Bob Zimmerman's, and Cricket's . . . and reflect on how each of them might have responded to the news . . . whether it could have been related better. Sarah strolls in. "What's up?" she says.

Ellen and I try to fashion our faces into pictures of unadulterated good news. Sarah sees right through us. "Was that Pai? What'd she say?"

We tell her. We pull no punches.

How she handles the news makes me feel so proud. She admits to still being worried. "It's scary knowing something that could kill me was inside of me, growing." But her worries she's husbanded into perspective. "I'm happy to put an end to the mystery, the 'suspected' this and that. I also now get it: why Dr. Pai was reluctant to do the surgery. I mean, if she hadn't found any cancer, I would have wondered, Was it worth it? Did I do the right thing? God's blessed me in that it was found early—thanks to Mom and doctors like Tanen to find it and Pai to remove it once it was found."


## MAY 29


With Sarah on the mend, we try to pick up the other pieces of our lives that had been put on hold. I return from a business trip to a text from Cricket: *plz call asap*.

I call her. "Hi. I've missed seeing you. What's up?"

"Hospice has given Daddy only a few days." Howard's cascading health problems have apparently reached the tipping point. He's contracted some sort of infection. They've pumped him full of antibiotics, but they're ineffective. "Daddy can't fight no more. He has no appetite. He's wasting away."

"Be right over."

Sarah overhears my conversation, and eyes me. She doesn't need to say anything, nor do I. But I want to. "Don't even try," she says. Still on the mend, I'm not sure she should join me. But she's sure.

We hop in my car, drive an hour, and show up at the Coopers' new place. Once evicted from their free trailer, a relative takes them in. As they're now so much further from me, I'm not able to see them as often as I'd like. I still manage a couple dozen visits, supplementing a new companion caregiver, who lives a lot closer. My visits make clear to me that, compared to their new set-up, the tiny jam-packed trailer was the Taj Mahal. Howard and Cricket miss it sorely.

At first, Sarah and I sit out on the back deck, with Cricket and her niece Bernice, up from North Carolina. Cricket sits, Bernice stands, both puff away. Maybe half the smoke dissipates or drifts into the woods abutting the house. The rest burns my eyes and Sarah's recently operated-on throat. But we don't say a word or give off any negative vibes.

Cricket updates Sarah and me on Howard's situation. It's grave. We express our condolences. Then, a thought popping into her head, Cricket sets down her cigarette and (as the smoke makes a beeline for my eyes and Sarah's throat) hops out of her chair to retrieve two large posters she's made: one for her, another for Howard. Each is a photomontage, reflecting their respective personalities. Howard's photos include one of him enveloped by kids on his lap, clinging to his shoulders, at his feet, another of him walking back from a favorite fishing hole, proudly hoisting a brace of bass. Cricket's include one of her at age five, in a red, spangled cowgirl outfit, another in a bikini.

"How old were you then?" I ask, pointing at the scanty swimsuit.

"Twenty. Maybe twenty-one. Sarah's age."

"You were really pretty," says Sarah.

"A heart breaker, more like it!" I say.

Cricket laughs, then, after a spell of coughing: "I got me some attention."

At an appropriate moment, Sarah says, "I just wanted to thank you, for all your help, in what I went through. For taking me shooting, helping me relax, putting things in perspective. It really helped, a lot."

"You're welcome, sweetie," replies Cricket, before taking a big drag. "How are things with you? Your dad tells me it all went well."

"Yes. It did. It was cancer. They are, they say, as near certain as they can be that they got it all and it won't come back."

"Your dad told me you don't need to go for radiation or chemo. That right?"

Sarah nods. "I'm so, so lucky."

I turn to Bernice. "I'm really sorry about your mom." Cricket's sister in North Carolina is also battling cancer. She's not so lucky. It's stage 4.

"Thank you."

"Excuse us for a moment, ladies?" I say to Cricket and Bernice as I flip Sarah a head nod and she follows me into Mr. Cooper's room. I pause in the hallway. "Just say 'hey,' then I'll give you a signal, you return to Cricket, and I'll stay a bit longer with Howard." Sarah nods.

Upon entering, I'm reminded of Dolly. The last time I saw her was the only time I'd ever seen her in bed; likewise, this is the first time I've ever seen him in bed, too. And, like Dolly was at the very end, Howard, too, is really struggling, similarly trying so hard not to let on that he's even worried, let alone suffering, as if even acknowledging his pain—or terror—would violate his deep-seated sense of etiquette, of being a proper host, the brave patriarch everyone's always looked to—like in the photo montage. But even this incredibly courageous, impeccably mannered man can't hide the pain. Each time he moves a millimeter, the catheter digs into his private parts. Uncontrollable wincing contorts his pale, pasty face. His dry lips are pocked with splotchy sores in various stages of blistering. Yet he bravely, politely dissembles. After I tell him I'm here with Sarah (for he can't see us), he ignores his situation, saying, "Hello, Sarah! How are you doing? How you doing, Eric? How are your parents?"

Sarah eyes me, and I nod. "Hello, Mr. Cooper. So nice to finally meet you. My dad talks about you all the time." She eyes me again, and I nod again. "I'm going to head back outside to be with Cricket. But I did want to meet you and say how much help Cricket was to me. So, thank you for being her father . . . such a good father, too."

"Perfect," I mouth.

"She said she had a good time with you, Sarah. Thank you for stopping by."

Once Sarah's gone, I say, "Everyone's good, Mr. Cooper. Thank you for asking." I, too, shower praise on Cricket. "She helped Sarah so much with her cancer—through the barrel of a forty-four mag extra-long."

This image makes him smile: of his tiny girl with her massive pistol drilling a bull's-eye, besting all the young bucks. He struggles to keep his eyes open.

I pull the chair as close to Howard as I can get. I chitchat some more, but he's not very responsive. I know he's doped up, and I know he's exhausted. "I'm going to let you rest, Mr. Cooper. I'm so sorry you're having such a hard time."

"Oh, it'll get better in a few days."

## JUNE 3

Cricket texts me: *Daddy passed will u b pallbearer?*

I phone her at once. "I'm so sorry! And, of course, I'd be very, very honored to be one of your father's pallbearers."

At the service, when the funeral home's in-house Southern Baptist preacher steps up to the pulpit, I know what to expect: fire, brimstone, and Judgment Day. My mom was reared Southern Baptist. Her mom, with whom I lived for the first sixteen years of my life, never—and I do mean never—smiled in my presence.

But Howard gets the better of the preacher, posthumously, thanks to the details of his life, as summarized (in writing) by Cricket. The preacher begins stern-faced and somber. But gradually, as he recounts colorful episode after colorful episode, his rigid facial muscles relax, and he gives up all pretense of not seeing the humor in Howard's decidedly un-Baptist behavior. "At first, when Howard got his new truck, he let his daughters ride in the front. But then he got King, his German shepherd. After that, the girls always rode in the bed. At the family pig roasts, it was always Howard tending the spit. He had a simple rule when pouring the rum he used to baste the pig. It was 'One for the hog, one for me.'"

But during the service laughter is muted because bruised egos defy interment and the surviving siblings have already turned from the shared, joyous memories of their father to the scabrous, jealous memories of their petty squabbles. Howard's death caused a great rift to form—re-form, actually—between two of his three surviving children: Cricket and her sister, and their respective clans. There aren't many people in attendance, they're mostly family, but this might as well be a mixed Serbian-Croat service, what with the silent stony distance separating the warring factions, the pews their Balkans.

Outside the funeral home, I join five other men in hoisting Howard's casket. It's my first time being a pallbearer, and, like the others, I don't want to screw things up. The casket's not so heavy, what with six pretty big guys doing the lifting. The key is the orchestration: out the funeral home door, down the steps, backing up into the hearse, and sliding the casket in—without skinning a knuckle or breaking a fingernail, let alone dropping Howard.

At the gravesite, the two factions veer off into different quadrants of tent and grass while the preacher quotes Jesus on love and forgiveness. In tribute to Howard's being a Seabee, the burial concludes with a twenty-one-gun salute. The spiffiness of the attire and synchronicity of the shots by three VFW riflemen aren't quite up to the standards of Arlington National Cemetery.

When things reconvene at the teetotaling wake at Front Royal's Baptist Tabernacle, only one faction shows up: Cricket's. She's bald, hoarse, skin and bones. Everyone hovers around her, trying to get her to eat and to believe that things will get better. None of us actually believes things will get better, but we lie with pure hearts.

It's then that I learn that, as incomprehensible as it sounds, the very day that Howard died, the sister who'd taken in Howard and Cricket when they were booted from the mobile home—evicted her sister. So, once again, the cancer-ridden Cricket finds herself a homeless, penniless nomad; this time turned out by her own kin.

It's not at all incomprehensible to Cricket, however. "My sister didn't agree with how I medicated Daddy. But I know what he wanted. She didn't. She couldn't accept my bucking her."

There is some good news, however. Bernice steps up and invites Cricket to come stay with her in North Carolina. This is especially generous, given the fact that Bernice's own mother (Cricket's other sister) is also battling stage 4 cancer.

But even this good fortune has a bittersweet aftertaste. "I wanted to die at home, in Virginia," says Cricket, picking at her fried chicken.

## JUNE 18

It's time to see Dr. Tanen again, for a follow-up. Of the tests Sarah will be getting every six months for the next few years, he says, "They're not going to find anything." He concurs with Drs. Ball and Pai, insisting that Sarah's life won't be impacted in any way. "Not in terms of years, and not in terms of quality of life."

## JUNE 30

Ellen, Sarah, and I embark for Hawaii to spend nearly six weeks on Kauai, with which we immediately fell in love four months prior, in February. Though excited, we know we must remain vigilant in using sunscreen to protect Sarah's scar.

## JULY 15

Two fat, animated Hawaiian monk seals waddle out of the surf up onto the beach, not ten yards from our place. When Ellen cries out, Sarah and I rush to the balcony of our second-floor lanai, and we all marvel. We go tell our next-door neighbor. "You've been coming here since sixty-nine," I say. "Have you ever seen anything like this before?"

"No," she says. "Never. They're nearly extinct. For two of them to just plop themselves down here, right in front of you, is, well, just incredible! You guys must be blessed!"

"We are indeed."

## AUGUST 7–9

During our last night on Kauai, we dine at Sarah's favorite spot, Calypso, where the servers are nice, the fish tacos are great, the frozen daiquiris are big, and the guys are cute.

Earlier in the day, I'd received a text. I'm not sure whether to share it here, now, but I do. In retrospect, my *Do* should have been a *Don't*.

"Bernice texted me earlier today," I say to Sarah. "Remember her? Cricket's niece?"

"Sure."

"Well . . . it's bad news, I'm afraid. Cricket died. Yesterday."

Sarah sets her taco down, looks at her plate, and starts to cry. "Excuse me." She rushes to the ladies room, while I feel like a heartless idiot.

Ellen's throat thickens. "I never even met her, but I feel like crying, too."

En route back from Hawaii, we stop off to see Matt, who's driven down from the place he's renting in California's Central Valley, which is near the vacant site of Little One's birth tepee. We have a blast, cursing at the confusing, pretzeling highways, rude drivers, and noisome smog, while chortling at the orange tans, implanted boobs, and incessant F-bombs out of the mouths of babes.

# WELCOME BACK

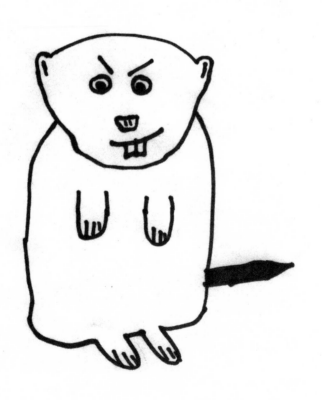

# DOs AND DON'Ts

**M**y companion caregiving began with a set of *Dos* and *Don'ts*, so perhaps it's a fitting way to conclude writing about it. Being just one unskilled guy with a set of very limited experiences, I'm reluctant to offer any sweeping suggestions. But here goes . . .

*Do embrace the power of hope.* All hospice patients are expected to be buried within six months, yet 17 percent are discharged—alive, many well. What gives? What gives is The Hoover of Hope. (Physicist David Bohm prefers "The Quantum Vacuum.") Use your Hoover to vacuum up all that depressing Dark Matter and Energy out there, so as to expose the Light. The way may at times seem—and be—narrow, but as illuminated by Bob, Dolly, and many others: the more patients exhibit hope, the longer they live and the happier they are. Ivy League cosmologists admit that only 4 percent of the universe is comprised of stuff we can observe directly; 96 percent can only be inferred by, for instance, the gravitational pull exhibited by the Dark stuff. Hope's gravitational pull is awesome. Sorbonne philosophers still sing the praises of René Descartes and his four-hundred-year-old hypothesis: "I think, therefore I am." But I find much more interesting—and practical—what two University of Rochester researchers hypothesized forty years ago when they coined the term *psychoneuroimmunology*: I hope, therefore I heal.

The Rochester thesis is well supported by studies at NIH, Harvard, Stanford, and through Faraday cage barriers. Though researchers may have finally "scientifically proven" that the brain and immune system comprise an integrated health system that can be tapped to ward off— or ameliorate—all sorts of ailments, to me this is nothing but a coat of academic varnish atop what dawned on humanity no later than the Axial Age, given voice much later in our Cenozoic Era by poets like Emily Dickinson and philosophers like Abraham Heschel. To wit, intentionality is a force to be reckoned with. So I say, Dismiss all those naysayers who dismiss your hopes as "wishful thinking." Embrace such thinking! Go with the flow of hope's gravitational pull!

*Do look for pontoons across the choppy seas of life.* John Donne ("No man is an island") was right: propitious quantum entanglements are everywhere, just waiting to be leveraged. From my first official hospice patient, Bob, to my last, Cricket, I've been astounded by the presence of so many latent, helpful connections, such as how Bob's bum eye helped me see better and how Cricket's battle with cancer helped my daughter cope with hers. I'm no linguist, but *hope* and *hospice* share more in common than just four letters.

*Do differentiate the connections*, however, such as by getting a truly independent second opinion. Doctors protect their own. (Being a lawyer, I can't blame them for circling the wagons.) Consequently, Doctor X will often recommend Doctor Y, and vice versa. However, this is not the way to go about getting a second opinion. Instead, reach out to friends, family. I realize that few people have best friends who are chaired professors and tops-in-their-field doctors at Johns Hopkins, but my guess is that most people, if they cast a wide-enough net, can locate someone able to render a truly objective second opinion. Furthermore, while online advice can be very helpful, if it's anonymous, as much is, take it with a grain of salt. Many "review sites" are replete with phony praise and ax-grinding criticism. Also, look not just for a second opinion but a second approach. Doctors Tanen and Ball are very different in their training, temperament, and professional foci. This divergence led to disagreements, such as regarding the merits of genetic testing, given the propensity for false negatives. However, they're both brilliant, compassionate men who recommended an equally brilliant woman: Dr. Pai.

When you find this sort of sweet spot bridging different approaches, it's often a very sturdy bridge.

*Do be vigilant regarding what you ingest.* For instance, my wife's research uncovered many problems with soybeans, which are in just about every processed or packaged food in the United States. Moreover, even "natural, organic soybeans" are problematic: studies show they interfere with the proper functioning of the thyroid gland and inhibit the absorption of thyroid medication. Mother Nature's fecund soil yields toadstools as well as truffles. That doesn't mean She intended us to stick them both in our mouth.

*Do get tested early and often.* Testing can be expensive, irritating, inconvenient. It can yield false positives or negatives. Nonetheless, I'm a big believer in testing, from full-spectrum bloodwork to annual sonograms. Even "big problems"—if caught early—can often be resolved with a minimum of cost and repercussions. By the same token, "small problems"—left undetected—can kill.

*Do realize that sunsets are best enjoyed outdoors.* The thing many of my patients most enjoyed doing was also the simplest and cheapest: enjoying the great outdoors. For instance, Howard, blind though he was, derived so much pleasure from opening the window in order to feel the breeze, smell the fresh-cut grass, and hear the birdsong. Cricket loved blowing her own puffs of cigarette smoke up toward the cotton-candy cumulous clouds.

*Don't let student-doctors test their training wheels on your loved ones.* Many American hospitals are teaching institutions. This means that the hospital serves two masters: the individual patient and the medical profession. This is not a bad thing, conceptually. It's noble and necessary. The only way students can really learn, after all, is through trial and error. However, there's a time for trial and a time for error. When your loved one's life is on the line, be alert to an inordinate amount of student involvement. Michelangelo had students, too, but he didn't let them chip away at the hunk of marble as he worked on David. Say to your doc, "Be like Mike."

Finally, in the words of the Prophet Isaiah (58:7): *"Don't ignore your kin."* Family members are often in need of companionship. If you're like me, you sometimes fail to recognize such needs—and opportunities.

## NOVEMBER 20, 2012

I'm spending less time with strangers, more with my loved ones. As my Chicago B-school finance professor might say, I've reallocated my most valuable asset—time. I've not abandoned hospice altogether. I still grab the occasional lunch with Bob Zimmerman's brother and Little One's adopted son, still visit Gordon's widow twice a month (travel and family emergencies permitting).

I inform Mara that I'm taking a "quasi-sabbatical" from hospice. "I love it!" she exclaims. "It's like *The Wizard of Oz*! You're looking for something, yet it's been right there in front of you, all along!"

My father's sure been right in front of me, giving Job a run for his money. Over the past few months he's suffered a mini-stroke, undergone emergency melanoma surgery, endured an esophageal ulcer and gastric bleed out (requiring an emergency four-pint transfusion), fallen and fractured his pelvis, and battled several infections, including a strange new virus to hit D.C.-area seniors. My dad's on a first-name basis at three hospitals. When he's not being wheeled into one, my mom often is.

## JUNE 10, 2013

Life is good. My parents have enjoyed a long stretch of mostly good health. (They deserve it!) My wife's juggling tennis, therapeutic riding, and all the stuff related to our kids that never even crosses my mind. Matt's begun hiking the Appalachian Trail in its entirety (2,175 miles), starting in Maine, while Sarah's begun working for a boutique provider of auxiliary legal services, her initial months to be split between D.C. and New York. (Her cancer's left her with a faint scar and a nightmare every now and again but also hard-won wisdom. She overhauled her eating and drinking habits and wrote her senior thesis at GW on the many ways nutrition can hurt—or help—one's quality of life and life expectancy.)

Given my limited skill set and experiences, I know there's only so much I can offer regarding hospice advice, tips, *Dos*, and *Don't*s. However, the world over, there are millions of experiences, from sons and daughters to nurses and priests, to some brave soul in Virginia who, battling ovarian cancer, nearing the end of her six-month ordeal, would like to help a terrified patient in Oregon who's just been informed she's also got six months, tops. I hope www.hospicevoices.com develops into an active—and interactive—forum for just this sort of sharing of best practices.

Take Mark Joseph's "Atonement Eulogy." Like many super-successful, super-busy sons, Mark didn't spend as much time as he would have liked with his father, George. (Sometimes I'd lunch alone with George because Mark was tied up in traffic or on a conference call with his Paris headquarters.) However, all's well that ends well, and Mark ended his relationship with George incredibly well, by reading his proposed eulogy to the one about to be eulogized. "Why shouldn't the most important audience member hear what I'm going to say?" asks Mark. "Plus, if my father were to want me to change anything, of course I want to." Mark assures his dad that—no matter how it may have appeared, no matter how dusty the mantel might have become—George never left the pedestal. Mark had always aspired to be like George: as good a family man, businessman, and community leader. In just a few minutes, every missed lunch, cut-short phone call, cross word, and bruised emotion—vanishes.

My father turned eight-seven today. My present to him was my atonement eulogy.

It took some time to unwrap.

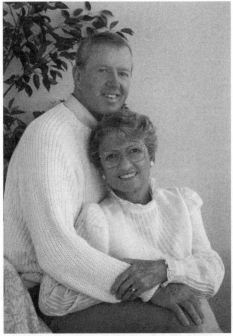

© Dale Kirk

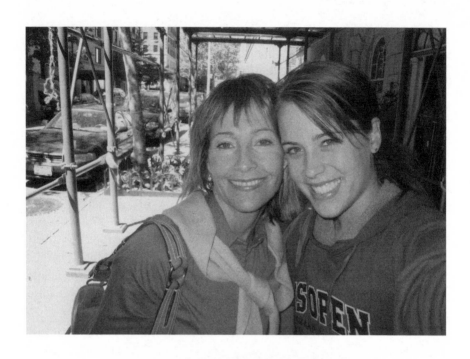

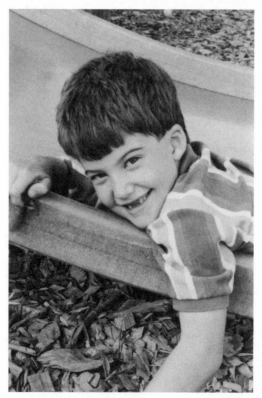

# ACKNOWLEDGMENTS

I'd suffer permanent insomnia were I not to credit certain people, without whom this book would not have been possible. I must start with my wife. Ellen Murray took a big chance in 1986, flying over from the Canary Islands to join forces with a crazy man. Ever since, she's been my rudder: an amazingly wise, supportive, and pragmatic partner, mother, and muse, let alone gorgeous.

However, a ship can't make much progress with just a rudder. That's where my kids come in. Years ago, I never gave much thought to having children. Now, I couldn't imagine my life without Sarah and Matthew. Their passion fills my sails.

My parents, Mary Jean and Thaddeus, have given me so much, from the love of books to material comfort (thanks to their hard work) to an appreciation for the psychic returns available via investments in community service. Other family members have also been very supportive.

The Rowman & Littlefield Publishing Group's gifted (and dogged) senior editor Suzanne Staszak-Silva had the vision to see (and courage to commit to) a book amid my mess of a draft manuscript. My superlative freelance writing coach Alexandra Shelley sharpened this vision into a narrative, anchored my plot, and refused to allow me to drift off-course. Neil Cotterill designed the wonderful cover. Meanwhile, Julia Loy and so many other fine folks at Rowman have had to contend with my many delays and miscellaneous nonsense. The linchpin has been Jed Lyons, Rowman's president and CEO. For years, his support and encouragement never drifted, never wavered. It's been a blessing and an honor having such talent backing me, rooting me on, patiently correcting my manifold failings.

So many books, far better than this one, haven't sold so well. If mine suffers a similar fate: my bad. If not, then it's largely due to the efforts of an extraordinary publicity and social media team. Here again it starts with Rowman, in the person of Rome marathoner Sam Caggiula. It also includes the wonderful Justin Loeber (and his fellow vocal cords at Mouth Public Relations: Patrick Paris, Hugh McIntyre, and Cassie Berwick), the irrepressible insomniac Susie Stangland, and my wise, lovely consiglieri, Lucinda Dyer. I owe a final, special debt of gratitude to the incredibly talented and scarily energetic Lee Woodruff, who, despite not knowing me from Adam and being crazy-busy, took an interest in this topic and book and allowed me to perform a Vulcan mind-meld on her mad skills.

Unfortunately I can't acknowledge all of the friends who endured my early, puerile drivel, rooted me on, or otherwise helped make this book a reality, but I must at least thank Paul Adkins, Richard Badger, Roger Blumenthal, Chris and Debra Brown, Shep Burr, Ken Cera, Bob Chernak, Jim Davis, Chris Davitt, Christine Ekman, Pat and Leon Eggers, Mike Faber, Christine Hazel, Aaron Iverson, Steve Jakubowski, Mark Joseph, Jeff Kleinman, Nelson Lund, Blythe Lyons, J. D. Mack, Retta and Warren Nowlin, Kim and Mark Pacala, Michael Peller, Wendy Post, Bill Ritchie, Kathy Roach, Sam Stopak, Holly and Tony Tedeschi, Liz and Jim Underhill, Bob Wenger, Bryan Wethington, and Joe Zell.

Last but quite clearly not least, I can't thank enough, or often enough, the extended Zimmerman, Hensley, Ford, Graziano, Burris, and Cooper families. By inviting me into their lives they revealed a richness of living—at the end of life—that I hadn't a clue existed. It's been a privilege knowing them and sharing their stories.

# ABOUT THE AUTHOR

**Eric Lindner** is an attorney and entrepreneur. A hospice volunteer since 2009, he divides his time between Warrenton, Virginia, and Kauai, Hawaii.